Contents

STEVEN SHAW & ARMAND D'ANGOUR

The Art
of Swimming

IN A NEW DIRECTION WITH
The Alexander Technique

Foreword by
VICTORIA WOOD

with illustrations by Julian Warner
and photographs by Jill McArthur

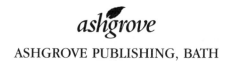

ASHGROVE PUBLISHING, BATH

Published by Ashgrove Press Limited
Bath Road, Norton St. Philip, Bath BA3 6LW, UK

First published 1996
Reprinted 1996

A CIP catalogue record for this book is held
by the British Library

ISBN 1-85398-095 1

*This book was designed and typeset
by Martyn James*

The front cover picture shows
Limor and Steven Shaw gliding under water,
photographed by Peter Rowlands of Ocean Optics

Printed in Great Britain by Redwood Books
Trowbridge, Wiltshire

Acknowledgements

This book became a much larger project than we originally imagined it would be, and we are grateful to all the individuals who freely lent their time and energy to help create it. Our publisher Robin Campbell steered us towards the title; friends scrutinised the original drafts for readability and the final proofs for errors.

Particular thanks are due to those who made valuable suggestions and comments at the initial stages: Georgina Evans, Denyse Faulkner, and Dr. Nina Meyer. Thanks also to all who kindly gave their time and permission to be photographed in or out of the water: Helen and Laura Allen, George Blair, Lea Clark, Eileen Emmerton, Odyssée Gaveau, Jamie Gayle, Tomoe Inoue, Angus McArthur, Ken McMullen, Rita Shamia, Robert Smith, and Oliver Suralli. We would also like to thank the large number of students and teachers who participated enthusiastically in our classes and talks and contributed to our ideas.

A number of experts in different fields have offered useful advice and encouragement: we would like to thank in particular Terry Laughlin, Dr. Chloë Stallibrass, and Deborah Taylor of Cassell. We are grateful for the practical help and suggestions of Sarah Barnet, Sharon Berry, Adam Jackson, Sue Trewin, and Simon Trewin of Sheil Land Associates; and for the supportive words of Dr. Laurence Gerlis.

The photographs and illustrations so crucial to this book are due mainly to the skill and tireless efforts of Jill McArthur and Julian Warner, both of whom went far beyond the call of duty in cheerfully lending their assistance to the project. We wish them the success they truly deserve. Thanks also to Walter Carrington, Horace Dobbs, Jane Goss (Picture Editor, The Telegraph), Edna Perlman, and underwater photographer Peter Rowlands (Ocean Optics), for providing some indispensable images. Gratitude is due to Andrew Barker and John Lyras (together with the staff of the Laboratory

Health Club, Muswell Hill) for their consistently generous support of the project, and for providing images and facilities for photography. Ken McMullen, who showed consistent support and enthusiasm for the project from its early stages, generously offered us the use of his floating studio on the Thames for the book-launch.

Victoria Wood, whose 4-year old son Henry already feels at home in the water, delighted us by readily agreeing to write her witty Foreword to the book. We much appreciate her gesture. She expresses, in her inimitable way, feelings that many swimmers will readily identify with.

Finally, we thank our respective partners and families for their advice, patience and support: Limor and the children, Talya and Tomer; and Karen.

Steven Shaw and Armand D'Angour
London, June 1996

Picture Credits

Jill McArthur (photography) has created award-winning photographic images of women for the *Sunday Times* colour supplement. She is particularly interested in photographing the human body in all its aspects.

Julian Warner (illustrations and cartoons) is a fine artist who lives and works in London. He is a freelance anatomical draughtsman and illustrator, and an assistant swimming instructor to Steven Shaw, with whom he studies the Alexander Technique.

Fig 1.3, p.23 (*F.M. Alexander*): Walter Carrington.

Fig 2.1, p.43 (*Laboratory Health Club*): © Telegraph Colour Library.

Fig 2.4, p.49 (*Nick Gillingham*), photo Anton Want: © Allsport Picture Agency.

Fig 3.1, p.67 (*Milingimbi, Australia*): © Axel Poignant Archive.

Fig 3.2b, p.68 (*Baby*): © Jessica Johnson.

Fig 3.11, p.88 and back cover (*Dolphin with man*): © Horace Dobbs.

Fig 4.4, p.95 (*Carl Lewis, Andrew Jameson*), photos David Cannon, Bob Martin: © Allsport Picture Agency.

Fig 4.10, p.104 (*Swimmer*), photo Simon Bruty: © Allsport Picture Agency.

Fig 5.4a, p.131 (*Turkana woman, Kenya*), photo L. Rudolf: © Royal Geographical Society.

Fig 5.4b, p.132 (*Sit-ups*): © Telegraph Colour Library.

Fig 5.9, p.142 (*Henry Mathers*), photo Bob Martin: © Allsport Picture Agency.

Fig 6.1, p.151 (*Ganges*): © Bipinchandra J. Mistry.

Foreword by

Victoria Wood

I was taught to swim at the age of ten in Bury Baths in Lancashire by a woman holding a pole and shouting. I could do a length of strained breast stroke and I could also do what was described on my certificate as a 'Simple Dive'. Really it was more of a panicked flop.

At secondary school I swam once a week. I loved the water but I never felt at ease in it. We spent a lot of time diving for bricks and treading water in our pyjamas, obviously readying ourselves for some incident similar to the sinking of the Titanic. A big annual highlight was the Swimming Gala, where we waited eagerly for the Long Plunge. This was invariably won by an enormous girl in a pink chequered costume, who floated interminably like a piece of living Battenburg.

In my twenties I would sometimes pootle about in a grubby, old-fashioned pool, but mainly I just fantasised about exercise, and didn't do any. I tried a thing that fastened to the doorknob that was supposed to give you a stomach like an ironing board, but I lost enthusiasm when someone opened the door and concussed me.

I started to swim again. I worked up from two lengths to twenty, and painfully did twenty lengths every time I went to a pool. I did that terrible contorted breast stroke you see so often, head half out of the water, spine scrunched up, eyes fixed desperately on the clock, praying for 'getting out time'.

Then a friend taught me how to do the breathing for crawl, and I loved the feel of that once I got the knack. I bought goggles and a racing costume, which were a great improvement. It meant I could swim without getting sore eyes or whacking an old age pensioner in the eye with an escaping bosom. I upgraded myself to forty

9

lengths and did it every weekday for about two years. Doggedly, and never showing any improvement, I did a 35 mile round trip, with forty lengths in the middle of it, day after day.

Of course, it became mind-numbingly boring, apart from the other disadvantages like always stinking of chlorine, and going around for part of the day with someone's old corn plaster stuck on my elbow. I would plough up and down, always doing crawl, because that was all I was comfortable with, never varying the routine. I would sometimes try and increase the pace, and would thrash harder and kick faster and yet not move through the water any quicker.

So I gave up on swimming. I did aerobics and weights and rubber bands and step and found that exercise could go hand in hand with enjoyment. But always, nagging at the back of my mind, was this feeling that I should be able to swim for fitness; and that if only I was told properly what to do, I would be able to get the joy that should be there for us when we're in the water.

I would love to be able to move through that element with the confidence I have when exercising on land. I do see now that that deadly, unvarying forty lengths is not a good, effective or enjoyable way to exercise. There are a lot of people, like me, who know enough to swim but not enough to hold themselves correctly or train effectively for everyday fitness. Although I already knew Steven because he teaches one of my children swimming, I can honestly say that this book is one I would have bought anyway. I want to know how to move in the water in the right way. I want swimming to be a joy and not a chore or a penance. I want wet fun, and if this book doesn't help me get it then I'm popping on my chequered swimming costume and going out for a Long Plunge.

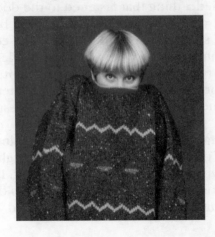

Authors' Foreword

The authority of those who teach is often an obstacle to those who want to learn.

Cicero

Steven Shaw

This book harmonises the perspective of two people who came to swimming from opposite ends of the spectrum. My co-author, despite a brilliant academic career at Eton and Oxford, had never learned to swim, and in his mid-30s was resigned to being a non-swimmer. Swimming lessons in his youth had been disastrously unsuccessful, and all subsequent attempts to learn had been a failure. He had looked for a book that would help him understand why he should want to swim as well as how – in other words to inspire him to learn. But no such book existed, which was when he first had the idea of writing it himself.

At that point he came to me for swimming lessons. Familiar with the Alexander Technique from his musical training, he was intrigued by the fact that I was both a swimming teacher and an Alexander teacher. The results were spectacular: he learned to swim in just a few weeks. A year on, he's a keen swimmer (and a qualified swimming instructor) and has shared his enthusiasm by helping teach children and adults to discover the joy of swimming for themselves. My application of the Technique in teaching swimming was instinctive and all-embracing, but largely unspoken. In fact, I myself had all but given up swimming until I started training to teach the Alexander Technique. In my youth I had become deeply involved in competition swimming. The discipline of training for hours every day dominated my early teens, and the desire to excel at the sport by swimming faster and faster became an obsession.

This took its toll: by the age of 17, swimming bored and exhausted me, and I gave it up altogether.

When I started training with the Alexander Technique, my teacher Zeev Tadmore suggested that my years of swimming were the main cause of stiffness in my upper torso. I started going to the pool to discover how this might have come about. The right sort of feedback is invaluable: I was lucky to have the help of my wife Limor, herself a swimmer and Alexander teacher. Thanks to her keen observation I became aware of the damaging efforts I exerted in pulling my head back in the breast stroke (my favoured stroke). I also noted that my competitive instincts were so ingrained that I couldn't let myself be overtaken, but would strain to stay ahead of other swimmers at all costs! Learning to check these habits and 'slow down' presented the challenge of discovering a new kind of self-control. It opened up for me an exciting new dimension, a sense of continuing exploration of the water and of myself.

Armand saw that the Alexander Technique could offer a useful perspective on learning to swim at any level, so I suggested to him that we collaborate in writing this book. His understanding of the obstacles which confront the learner, and his skill at articulating the connections between swimming and the Alexander Technique, helped deepen my appreciation of the complexities faced by all who seek to improve their ability in the water. Together we teased out the implications of how swimming with the Alexander Technique becomes more than *just* swimming: something worthy of being called the *art* of swimming.

Armand D'Angour

After being afraid of water most of my life, I never expected to learn to swim in my 30s. Doing so felt like a miraculous conversion. For years I had watched as others swam, jumped, dived and snorkelled. Everyone seemed to love the water, except me. I was unable to shake off my fear, and had nightmares about drowning. I had almost reached the stage where I thought I didn't even want to learn. Yet... an insidious pressure remained, particularly when I travelled in parts of the world which offered the prospect of clear, fresh lakes or calm blue seas: immensely enticing – if only I could allow myself to be enticed.[1]

Why should I want to swim? How could it help me? And how could I learn to overcome the fear? Surely there were others who felt the same, but like me couldn't get the answers from their swimming-teachers or find them in a book. So I thought I would write one myself. They say that if you want to learn something well, teach it. But a swimming-book written by a non-swimmer? *Chutzpah* aside, it makes sense. Adult non-swimmers have a valuable perspective on the obstacles they face in learning to swim, or even *wanting* to learn: things like fear of failure, uncertainties about breathing, worries about submerging one's face, the potential for panic and discomfort. I could look at all these things with eyes untainted by familiarity or expertise.

Even if Steven had not been an Alexander teacher, I expect he would still have taught me how to swim. But clearly his teaching methods and ideals were profoundly influenced by the principles of the Alexander Technique. Thoughtful and patient, he exuded a reassuring calmness and the absence of any sense of pressure to get results, which was exactly what was needed. He also understood the value of teaching adult beginners in a clean, well-heated swimming pool, with no threatening "deep end"and mercifully free of anxiety-inducing distractions. He differed from every other swimming teacher I had ever come across by taking nothing for granted.

This seems all the more surprising because, unlike me, Steven couldn't recall ever having been afraid of water. As a boy, he took to

---

[1] For too many people still, swimming is unfortunately associated either with overcrowded beaches and polluted seas, or with heavily chlorinated, unhygienic public pools, grubby changing-rooms, and dictatorial teachers. We hope that this book will help to promote continued awareness of the need both to provide sympathetic teaching and to preserve attractive environments for swimming.

the water with joy and ease. His story of how he came back to swimming via the Alexander Technique is a lesson in how important this approach might be for swimming teachers, competitive swimmers, and ex-competition swimmers, as well as for beginners of all ages.

Coming from two very different perspectives on water, our viewpoints are unified in this book by an appreciation of the valuable lessons that the Alexander Technique has to offer. I have not only benefited from Steven teaching me how to swim, but also from his energy and enthusiasm in working with me on this project. I doubt that I would have ever got round to writing *my* swimming book if it had not become *our* swimming book. Learning to enjoy water and rediscover the joy of swimming has been a transforming experience for us both, and we hope this book will inspire others to do the same.

Introduction

For art comes to you, proposing frankly to give nothing but the highest quality to your moments as they pass, and simply for those moments sake.

Walter Pater

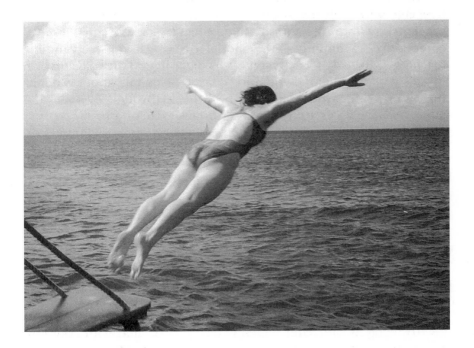

Can swimming be an *art*? In this book, we question the conventional view of swimming as a *sport* in which the prime requirements are fitness and skill, and where higher levels of competence may be attained through a focus on technique. Such an approach sets up pre-defined goals, in particular the attainment of speed. Swimming in a competitive context is about swimming fast, which involves knowing how to manoeuvre through the water with maximum efficiency. But at its best, the efficiency of a good swimmer's technique cannot be divorced from artistic style. It is elegant because it is effective, and it works because it is beautiful. Good swimming attracts praise for aesthetic qualities. Great swimmers – dolphins as well as Olympic medallists – are notable for qualities of gracefulness, flow and economy of movement. As in a great picture or piece of music, there is a sense of completeness about a lovely swimming style. Nothing seems out of place or redundant. The fine swimmer is a natural artist in the water.

Few handbooks exist that can inspire adults, whether swimmers or non-swimmers, to learn effective swimming skills. Instructional books tend to focus on methods for *swimming faster or further*, rather than on *swimming well and enjoying the water.* Furthermore, when technique is discussed it is often couched in language which, in the words of US coach Terry Laughlin, "makes efficient swimming sound like rocket science". High-level competitive swimming – the model on which most swimming teaching is based – is presented as fighting a battle against an intransigent opponent. Swimming coaches even talk about water as the "wall": one which can only be broken through by ease and guile, because it certainly cannot be attacked head-on.

Fighting with the water is one perspective. Many swimmers do it without realising it. But water will never allow us to do what it cannot do for us. Co-operating with it, exploring our relationship to it, understanding and valuing its qualities, can be the basis of a far more productive approach, one which we emphasise throughout this book. Whether water is to be treated as a hostile opponent or a generous ally is a matter for us to decide for ourselves. If we know how, we can derive marvellous benefits from its properties of buoyancy, fluidity, and density – the properties that allow us to float, to flow, and to swim.

Swimming is not just about manoeuvring oneself through the water. It is also about being *in* water and *with* water. There is an art just to being in the water which is rarely associated with common conceptions of swimming, and has much more to do with the *quality* of the experience. When swimming is approached as an art, rather than a technique, a science, or a means to fitness, it takes on a whole new dimension. First of all, the whole motivation for the swimmer changes. The emphasis is not on getting there faster, or on winning a race against other swimmers for a pre-ordained reward. Its significance becomes less narrow and more exploratory.

The reward is not an object presented at the end of a race, but is present in the very process of exploration and in the pleasure of enhanced awareness in the water.

Art involves skill, but occupies a wider domain than skill. Doing something with art means discovering the peculiar excellence appropriate to the activity. Whereas activities are often undertaken for narrow practical ends, art exists for an abundance of reasons and purposes. Its goals may be the imitation of nature, as in painting and sculpture, or the pursuit of beauty, rhythm, and harmony, as in music or poetry. The symbolic qualities of art overlap in different media: a picture can have rhythm just as can a dance, and music expresses moods and colours as does as a visual medium. Art is both self-expression and communication. It may involve the challenge of grappling with a physical medium to produce something that transcends pure physicality. Its deepest source is a part of our mind that does not reason, yet has a logic of its own. It has meanings that seek to be articulated but cannot be pinned down by words. Ultimately, art exists in itself and for itself.

How does the Alexander Technique encourage the swimmer to view swimming as an art? By giving us a closer understanding and appreciation of the working of the self. This awareness empowers us to think and act creatively, helping to set us free from the constraints of our automatic responses. As a result we can approach the water with a new sense of exploration, and discover a living, continuously unfolding relationship with it which goes beyond static, fixed ideas and conventional instruction. As our awareness is wakened to the way we move and function, we enter new realms of possibility for developing and exploring ourselves and our world. The Technique points us in the direction of thinking and acting in a freer, more balanced and integrated way – a key to the art of living itself.

A creative approach to the water is part of a creative approach to life. Age-old as well as new-age philosophies emphasise that truth is in the here and now. Too often, we grasp the kernel of this thought and twist it to derive tangible, egotistic profit from the truth it embodies. Yoga, for instance, is promoted as a way of getting fitter, slimmer, and stronger, and meditation is practised as a means to financial success, or to "win friends and influence people"! Whatever the validity of these aims, can we draw back from such a narrowly goal-oriented approach? Thoughtful interaction with the water offers a possibility, because it encourages us to drop the focus on cultivating our ego and compels us to accept a deeper, truer, less subjective reality. Water cannot be tamed. It doesn't care how fast we swim, how hard we try, or how badly we want to succeed. It ebbs, flows, and swells regardless. What it seems to do to us is a reflection of what we do to ourselves. It will support us if we let it, resist us if we fight it, and frighten us if we approach it with fear. It is unconquerable because it does nothing, seeks nothing, needs nothing – it just *is*.

This book follows the natural flow of ideas which connect the Alexander Technique with the swimmer's art. Chapter 1, *The Wakening of Awareness*, describes the origins and key principles of the Technique, and outlines how they can be applied to learning to swim. The second chapter explores how we view and perform fitness activities, and suggests an alternative approach: *Fitness Can Damage Your Health!* The third chapter tackles rarely addressed issues regarding psychological barriers to swimming, and indicates the positive path to being *At Home in the Water.* Chapters 4 and 5 plunge into core aspects of the Alexander Technique with crucial implications for the art of swimming: *Leading with the Head* and *The Art of Breathing.* The book concludes with reflections on water itself, celebrating the wondrous element that inspires the art of swimming and makes it possible: *In Praise of Water.*

1. The Wakening of Awareness

Self-knowledge is not a thing to be bought in books. Nor is it the outcome of a long, painful practice or discipline, but it is awareness from moment to moment of every thought and feeling as it arises.

Krishnamurti

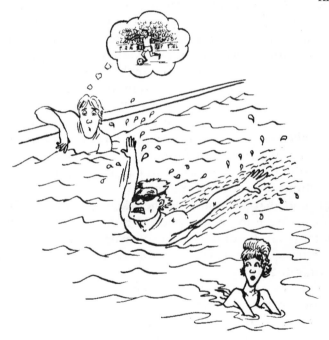

Fig 1.1 *At the pool.*

Just look at these swimmers: the bored expression, bared teeth, awkward paddle. Swimmers like this can be seen in every pool, every day of the week. Where are the carefree, elegant swimmers who obviously love the water and are such a pleasure to watch? They seem to be out of the frame. Is this what swimming is all about –

boredom, strain and discomfort? Non-swimmers can settle back in their chairs with a sigh of relief – they are obviously not missing anything. Yet...are you that non-swimmer? Or do you, perhaps, recognise something of yourself in any of these caricatures? There's a good chance, of course, that the very swimmers on whom these characters are modelled would not recognise themselves. In their different ways, they all exhibit a common feature: a lack of awareness of what they are actually doing.

We all know ways in which we limit our awareness. Awareness exists on different levels. There's awareness of the here and now, such as when we're doing something and enjoying every minute of it. Clearly not the experience of the figure on the left: his mind is on other things – the week-end, the ball-game – anything other than what he's actually doing. Secondly, there's the sort of awareness that depends on knowledge: knowing, for instance, how to use one's body in breast stroke, or why swimming with one's head stiffly out of the water is not a good idea. The young woman on the right of the picture obviously reckons that swimming is good exercise – so long as she keeps her hair dry! Then, there's awareness of the wider picture: understanding that all our actions are part of our life, and when our approach lacks balance, knowing how to redress it. The figure in the centre is all too familiar: jaw clenched, heedless of other swimmers, he strains his taut muscles against the water in an ungainly butterfly stroke, his sole aim to cut a half-second off his length. What more has he to learn? Everything, in our view, about the *art* of swimming.

It's often said that swimming is the ideal type of exercise, the best way of exercising the whole body in a medium where the risk of injury is minimal. It combines the pleasure of a sport with the benefits of fitness. But the fact remains that many people don't associate swimming with pleasure, and even those who swim out of choice seem to lack a sense of fun. They struggle through the water, their heads pulled back and their faces set in a grimace (Fig 1.2) their sole purpose simply to complete a fixed number of laps. They act as if the water were an assault course which must be battled through from a sense of duty, rather than for pleasure or profit. Unaware of how they appear to others, they even seem oblivious to the nature of their own experience. Regular swimmers persuade themselves that at least it's doing them good. But how much good can it do if their mind is elsewhere? If our mind isn't engaged in what we're doing, the benefits of exercise are limited or non-existent. What a waste of time if we can't even enjoy it.

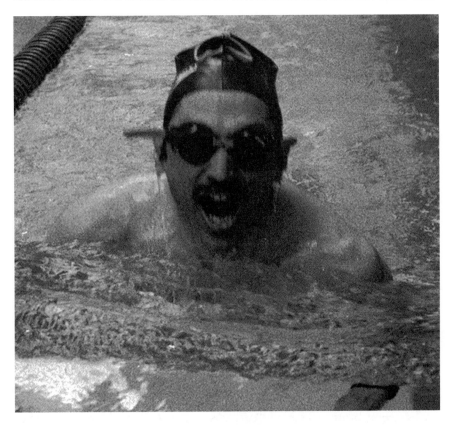

Fig 1.2 *No pain, no gain?*

Why is it that so many swimmers merely go through the motions rather than pay attention to the quality of their experience? Why don't we discover how to enjoy swimming more than we do? One reason is that enjoying the water is usually taken for granted in swimming teaching. Swimming instruction traditionally focusses on ways of moving the arms and legs, on techniques for swimming faster and longer, or on ploughing up and down a pool for extended periods of time. How we *think and feel* about swimming (and even *what* we think about when we swim) is generally ignored. But these aspects can be crucial – especially if our feelings are negative, as they often are. Fear, for instance, or boredom, which are feelings that many people associate with swimming, are rarely dealt with in a knowledgeable and constructive way. Yet such attitudes are widespread, and clearly have an important bearing on our relationship to the water.

For this reason, any approach to teaching swimming should give due attention to how we think and feel. If it doesn't, it overlooks the intimate connection between thought and action. Division of the physical and the mental is commonplace in our scientific age. But while it's hard to avoid talking about these domains as if they were quite separate, in doing so we create an artificial and harmful disunity. It gets in the way of resolving the difficulties we may have in learning how to perform activities which require physical skill, and allows teachers to neglect a valuable resource – the mind's ability to direct the body.

Many swimmers, for instance, don't realise that specific problems in swimming relate to unresolved anxieties. But it takes only a moment's consideration to realise that swimmers at all levels can be affected by such feelings, which are bound not only to detract from our ability to swim, but also to hinder the real potential for deriving pleasure from the water. Traditional swimming lessons train us to divorce our mental processes from the physical activity in hand – rather than, say, to make our fears explicit and to be educated to overcome their inevitable side-effects. In blocking out thoughts and feelings about what we are trying to learn, we deliberately approach the learning experience with less than total sensitivity. We thus obstruct a vital aspect of our organic mind-body awareness – in short, of our *self*.

Because brain and body processes are in fact inseparable, the way we think and feel in and about ourselves is the foundation for our development as swimmers. A truly effective approach to swimming should therefore begin by appreciating the unity of the self – which is the basis of the Alexander Technique. Built on the principle of developing *self-awareness in action*, the Technique is a system of *psychophysical re-education* – a means of increasing our control over the way we act and think. Applied to swimming, it starts by prompting us to an awareness of how our thoughts affect our actions in the water – an awareness which furnishes the swimmer with valuable tools for learning. It encourages us to discover our individual relationship to water, to find pleasure and to make real progress – not simply in terms of speed – in swimming. It indicates a direction both for improving our stroke and discovering new avenues to explore how water can be enjoyed. More broadly, it indicates a path of personal growth and empowerment. Swimming becomes not only a valuable activity to engage in with pleasure: as the *art* of swimming, it is a vehicle for bringing about renewed physical and emotional well-being, and for enhancing our lives through creative action.

The Alexander Technique Defined

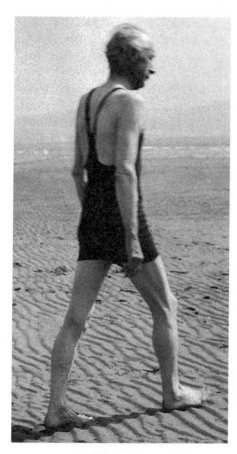

Fig 1.3

F.M. Alexander on the beach in his 70s, illustrating the qualities of good use to which he dedicated his life's work.

What is the Alexander Technique? Although it is becoming more widely known and practised, its essence is often misunderstood. It's not a form of relaxation treatment, massage, or a set of exercises designed to correct bad posture – although it is often used to reduce stress and improve posture. The Technique is primarily a method for teaching us to exercise conscious control over a particular set of reflexes, which are seen as the source of unproductive habits. The basic tendency is *to pull the head back and down*, either in response to an unpleasant stimulus, or simply because the movement has become an unconscious habit. The effect of this movement is to set in train a series of involuntary, and unhelpful, patterns of behaviour. Automatic physical reactions, with potentially negative effects on both mind and body, are not normally under our conscious control. They are habits which we fall into without thinking, unwittingly developed as a result of pressures imposed on us from infancy. They develop into a tendency to react to situations in ways over which we exercise limited conscious choice.

The Alexander Technique (abbreviated in this book to "the *AT*" or "the Technique") helps us to re-assert effective command over the way we think and act. It starts by making us aware of how a balanced relationship between the head and back can have an important influence on the body as a whole. It gives us a means of intervening to inhibit the actions that disturb this balance, and so provides a foundation for us to prevent the unhelpful patterns which arise in consequence. It has been described as "*un*learning the habits of a lifetime", habits which perpetuate an unhealthy fragmentation of the self. We invariably go wrong when we divorce our mental processes from our physical being. The *AT* is a practical method for putting us back in touch with our bodies, and thereby bringing about a psychophysical re-integration, which is particularly helpful in overcoming habits that impede the development of new skills. These principles are applicable to diverse activities in daily life: the *AT* is used in areas ranging from acting, riding, and golf to learning to play musical instruments and giving birth. The beneficial effects of the *AT* are widely recognised, and it is increasingly recommended by doctors as treatment for a range of ailments from stress to back pain.

Not only are unconscious habits an obstacle to mastering any creative activity, but they get in the way of enjoying the experience to the full. This is as true for swimming as for any other activity. Swimming can easily become boring if one ploughs through the water automatically, without any sense of development and exploration. Incorporating the *AT* brings the whole process to life. By opening ourselves to greater awareness through practising the Technique out of the water, we can discover in swimming a tremendous opportunity for continuing development and endless self-exploration. The following sections give an account of how the *AT* developed and how it is taught today, introducing some of its main concepts in **bold print**. It's worth becoming familiar with these terms: although some *AT* phrases have a Victorian ring (reflecting the era in which the Technique originated), its principles have far-reaching implications for the art of swimming that is the subject of this book.

How the Alexander Technique Developed

The story of how the Alexander Technique developed is worth telling both for its intrinsic interest and for the light it sheds on how it is practised today. Frederick Matthias Alexander, after whom the Technique is named, was born in Tasmania in 1869. He grew up in an environment which offered him a wealth of opportunity to observe nature. A youthful interest in animals helped him to develop a keen sensitivity to the way both animals and humans move and function. In his early twenties he moved to Sydney with a view to becoming an actor: in the 1890s there was a vogue for the performance of dramatic recitations, in which actors would declaim on stage passages from Shakespeare and other dramatists. Although he was successful as a stage performer, Alexander found to his dismay that during performances his voice often became hoarse. After one occasion when it failed completely he sought medical treatment, but despite rest and medication the loss of voice recurred when he returned to the stage.

Although he had suffered from respiratory problems from birth, Alexander was forced to realise that his vocal difficulties were not caused by a condition which could be treated by conventional medical means. They were a direct consequence of his reaction to the strain of performing. Something he was *doing to himself* – an unidentified physiological response to the conditions of performance – was causing him to lose his voice. To discover what was happening, he decided to find a way of observing himself while reciting. Using a structure of mirrors, he examined himself closely from different angles as he recreated the conditions of performing on stage. Over a long period of repeated self-observation he identified a particular movement which he invariably made as an involuntary reaction to stress: pulling his head *backwards and down*. The effect of this habitual action, he noted, was to alter the whole poise of his body, causing it to contract and stiffen. He gradually became convinced that this was the root of his problems. Amongst other things, it put severe pressure on his vocal mechanism, affecting his ability to breathe freely and to declaim.

Alexander became aware that the same reaction occurs in a wide variety of everyday activities, resulting in a degree of unnecessary tension in circumstances widely different from the stage. Pulling the head back and down is familiar as a defensive response in mammals, known as the **startle reflex**. It commonly occurs in the context of sudden fear or discomfort, the sort of conditions under which animals – and human beings – become immobilized or "freeze" (see Fig 1.4). Whatever its evolutionary purpose, it serves no useful function in everyday life. On the contrary, it tends to interfere with regular functioning. The tension it creates

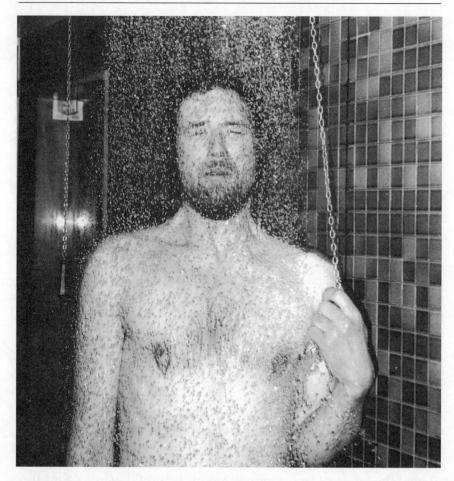

Fig 1.4

throughout the body reflects the effort of combating the alarm which triggers it. Retracting our head in this way becomes so habitual that we rarely notice when it happens. Alexander concluded that the solution to his difficulties lay in teaching himself to become aware of this reaction, and consciously intervening to stop it happening. He set out to discover how, with the right kind of preparation, he might find a way of deliberately refusing to allow himself to react to stimuli in an automatic way. His new approach centred on becoming more aware of the relationship and balance between his head, neck and back. He came to regard this relationship as fundamental in all activity, and for this reason termed it **the primary control.**

Although Alexander felt he had made an important discovery, the solution was not straightforward. He found that he constantly slipped back into habitual patterns without realising what was happening. Any attempt to reverse this by deliberately straightening up merely compounded his tension. He realised that it was important to eliminate any ill-conceived effort to "correct" his posture. The solution was not to be sought in purely physical terms – by using the muscles in a one-off corrective measure – but involved both mind and body acting continuously in concert. Observing the processes that caused the distortion of his poise, he devised a system for combining mental and physical responses in an integrated way. As he learned to prevent patterns of what he called **misuse**, his voice problems receded, and he noted coincidentally a considerable improvement in his general health: the breathing difficulties that had beset him from youth were cured. Resuming his acting career, he proceeded to apply his newly-acquired skills to improving his stage performances. The concepts of **use and misuse** were to become central in the Technique: the book in which Alexander himself describes how the method evolved is called *The Use of the Self.*

Although Alexander originally set out to find a solution to his own problems, he rapidly became aware of the same patterns of misuse in nearly everyone he encountered. He initially began to teach his Technique as a method for overcoming breathing problems. He gradually developed his characteristic teaching system, a combination of verbal guidance and gentle **direction** with his hands, which aimed to foster in his pupils a new sensitivity stemming from a better, freer **head-neck-back relationship**. Shortly after the turn of the century he moved to London, where he continued to develop and teach his Technique until his death in 1955. Through his methods, many individuals have learned to discover their own patterns of psychophysical **misuse** and to overcome them by bringing them under **conscious control**. The Alexander Technique not only provides important insights into how to enhance health, but is a method for getting in touch with ourselves. As such it has wider implications, akin to the philosophies of Zen and Yoga, as Alexander and other eminent adherents of his method (including the writers George Bernard Shaw and Aldous Huxley) were quick to realise.

The Alexander Technique in Practice

When an investigation comes to be made, it will be found that the very thing we are doing in the work is exactly what is being done in nature where the conditions are right – the difference being that we are learning to do it consciously.

F. M. Alexander

As babies and young children we possess a natural poise which enables us to move without undue strain or effort (see Fig 1.5). As we grow older we acquire greater muscular control of our limbs, but in the process we lose a degree of flexibility. Children are regularly told to 'stand up straight', 'walk properly', 'sit still'. In striving to comply, it's no wonder that we acquire ways of using ourselves which interfere with natural ease of movement. Even in apparently simple activities like sitting and standing we use redundant movements and unnecessary effort. Excessive tension accumulates and leads to physical strain, which can eventually result in specific symptoms such as headaches, sore backs, and frozen shoulders and necks. More generally, the strain shows itself in adults as stress, stiffness, and a lack of vitality and poise.

The Alexander Technique in practice tackles the source of these problems rather than the symptoms. Individual lessons are the norm. The teacher uses verbal suggestions and manual guidance to heighten the pupil's awareness of misuse: for instance, directing by gentle pressure of the hands to sit down or rise from a chair, to walk around the room, or to lie on a table while the teacher's hands impart a sense of **lengthening and widening** to the upper body. A deeper understanding of the Technique and its effects tends to emerge in the course of lessons rather than being directly taught. Through prompting of hand and voice, the teacher encourages the **release** of over-tensed muscles and helps to reactivate natural reflexes. These promote a sense of the upward **orientation** of the spine, allowing in turn an overall release of the musculo-skeletal structure, more relaxed and fuller breathing, and freer movement of the limbs.

Teaching the *AT* differs from most types of teaching in that there is no "right way" of doing it. The emphasis is actually taken away from trying to do the "right" thing, and instead attention is directed towards *eliminating the wrong*. When it comes to the workings of

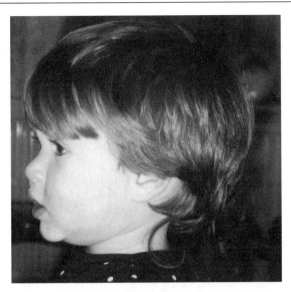

Fig 1.5
*A 2-year old child shows the poise
with which human beings are naturally endowed at birth.*

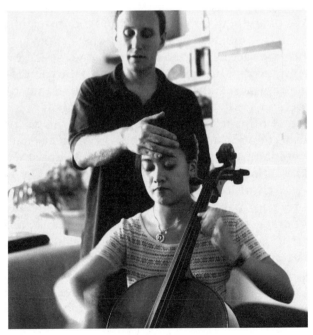

Fig 1.6
*Teaching the Alexander Technique: improving the
awareness of our performance.*

our own bodies, our senses are surprisingly unreliable. We generally have inaccurate ideas about exactly what we do when we
respond to stimuli such as a touch or a verbal instruction. F.M.
Alexander called this **faulty** (or **unreliable**) **sensory appreciation.**
It arises from unawareness of how we use our bodies, and is
compounded by the dulling effects of years of habitual misuse. It's
therefore important in learning the *AT* to understand that we
cannot rely exclusively on sensation. All we can do is to remain
open to the possibility of change.

Whilst a trained eye can spot what happens when we react in
our habitual fashion, our own senses are liable to give
inaccurate information about what we are actually doing. Long-
standing habits are so deeply ingrained that they have come to feel
normal, and any change, even for the better, may initially feel
wrong. Furthermore, when we actively *try* to bring about desired
changes, we are almost certain to make matters worse. The
inclination to try hard to achieve a given goal is, more often than
not, a major obstacle to progress in learning. F.M. Alexander
frequently cautioned against this attitude, which he called **end-
gaining**. Instead of focussing narrowly and unproductively on the
ultimate goal of any activity, we are encouraged instead to be aware
from moment to moment. This allows us to pay constructive
attention to the actual experience and the specific processes
involved in any action: in Alexander's term, to the **means-whereby.**

The *AT* emphasises that the muscles and frame of a living,
breathing person are in a condition of dynamic balance, constantly
on the move. For this reason, *AT* teachers *avoid* the word 'posture',
which tends to imply a static pose – the sort of misuse familiar from
images of soldiers on parade standing stiffly to attention. The
dynamic and mindful nature of the *AT* is brought out by its
description as **thinking in activity**. Specific conditions, such as
poor posture, back pain, or breathing difficulties, are viewed from
the overall perspective of *misuse*. As described above, misuse most
often occurs in connection with pulling the head back and down,
as in the startle reflex. This action has a detrimental effect on overall
functioning and leads to the build-up of strain. In the course of
lessons in the *AT*, the pupil gradually learns to be aware of this
reaction and to consciously prevent (or **inhibit**) it,[1] promoting

---

[1] The different connotations of "inhibit" should not be confused. F.M. Alexander
used the term to refer to forestalling the *habits* which interfere with good use.
Nowadays, due to Freudian associations, "inhibition" is commonly used to refer to
the suppression of painful *emotions*.

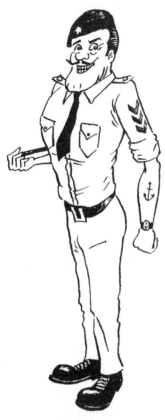

Fig 1.7
"Atten-SHUN!"

improvements in overall health and in the performance of everyday activities.

People who come to the *AT* suffering from specific ailments are often surprised that their problem is not focussed on directly. Modern medicine tends to treat different parts of our bodies in isolation. The highly-specialised medical approach does not encourage individuals to view themselves and their health in an integrated way. The *AT*, by contrast, is characterised by a holistic and non-direct approach to medical conditions. During lessons attention is not paid to parts of the body in isolation, but to the overall co-ordination and balance of the *whole* organism. The experience of *AT* students, as of Alexander himself, is that remarkable and sustained improvements in specific conditions can be made through bringing about the improved functioning of the organism as a whole.

Thinking in Activity

The initial lesson in learning the *AT* is to become *aware* of our habitual reactions and to apply the decision to *stop*. Once we have learned to prevent an unthinking reaction we can *choose* to apply a response based on reasoned judgement. Responding in this way requires us to attend to ourselves in the present moment. Stopping unthinking habits puts us in the position of being able to exercise choice rather than be subservient to unchecked automatic reactions. The radical difference between our normal patterns of behaviour and the process of **thinking in activity** can be illustrated by the following model (Fig 1.8). In this model we see how one pathway leads to a pattern of habitual reactions which result in a 'vicious spiral' of misuse, tension and pain. Conversely, by learning to break the habit, we enter into a 'virtuous spiral' of awareness and the freedom to act in a healthy way.

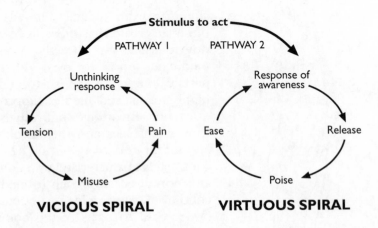

Fig 1.8

It's not easy to remain constantly alert to ourselves in this way! We are creatures of habit, and not used to the idea that we can renew our self-awareness from second to second. Inevitably, we find ourselves slipping back into habitual reactions and unthinking habits. However, through practice of the *AT* it becomes easier to notice the signals of misuse and to respond in an appropriate way.

Alexander frequently said that only by *stopping the wrong* can better use emerge, and in the *AT* great importance is attached to this principle. As the pupil progresses, understanding of what "stopping" entails matures and deepens. It doesn't mean doing nothing at all so that you collapse in a heap! It relates specifically to stopping the familiar, unwanted and unnecessary habits of our physical and mental responses. Only in this way can we recognise how habitual these patterns are, and be empowered to overcome them so that we can live our lives with a new and more creative awareness.

The Force of Habit

We get into the habit of living before acquiring the habit of thinking.

Albert Camus

Everything we do involves a complex interaction of conscious and unconscious actions. As we have shown, in practice the *AT* tends to work with relatively undemanding, commonplace activities, like standing, sitting, and walking. The effort of performing more complicated activities is likely to furnish distractions from the initial task at hand, that of learning to be aware of ourselves. Krishnamurti once remarked "There is more to life than getting in and out of a chair"! Similarly, there is more to playing the piano than just pressing the keys; but to be able to do so with the appropriate

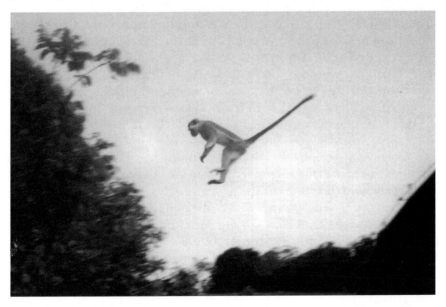

Fig 1.9
*Exhibiting perfect balance, a monkey leaps across
a wide gap with ease.*

amount of weight and balance is the foundation of all further learning of the instrument. In the same way, even sitting and standing with a new mindfulness can bring enormous benefit. It is the basis of a self-awareness that can be extended to any other activity.

Are you aware which sets of muscles you use when you get up from a chair? Logically, you may agree that the most efficient way of doing this would be to let your lower body – legs, hips and lower back – do most, if not all, of the work. But notice for yourself what happens when you begin to stand up. Do you find your neck or shoulders tensing? Are muscles in your upper body contracting?

The decision to rise from a chair is often accompanied by a contraction of neck muscles which pulls the head back. This is followed by an unnecessary downward pressure on the legs. These responses are so habitual that we don't notice ourselves making them. But are they necessary or desirable? The small backward movement of the head, clearly related to the 'startle reflex' mentioned above, creates a strain on the neck and a contraction of the spine. Put simply, we are *doing too much*. Note the lightness and grace of a cat jumping up onto a wall, or a monkey springing from a branch (Fig 1.9): because it is oriented upwards, it exerts the minimum necessary downward force. Its head and body function as an integrated unit. Similarly, what is needed for you to rise from your chair is for your body to be well oriented in an upward direction. All the relevant muscles are then engaged at the right moment, working together in harmony to take your body upwards. In this way, getting out of a chair requires a lot less effort than we normally use.

When we get up or sit down in our habitual, unthinking manner, the unnecessary muscular tension that we have engaged in our body and limbs persists. Our muscles stay taut, our spine remains contracted. Our body becomes effectively locked in a state of unnecessary strain, which in turn affects our thinking (the 'vicious spiral' of Fig 1.8). In subsequent actions – walking, driving, climbing stairs – we labour under the disadvantage of already lacking the basis for dynamic poise and flexibility. The constant repetition of such actions in the course of a day compounds the strain we unwittingly place on our musculo-skeletal structure, sapping us of freshness and vitality. The cumulative effects of **misuse** thus affect both bodily and mental functioning. No wonder most people feel drained at the end of a working day.

By proposing that we direct attention to the starting-point of the tension at the top of the spine (sometimes referred to as the *sub-occipital* or *atlanto-occipital* joint) – the *AT* proposes a practical way in which we can become, and remain, alert to ourselves. In the *AT* session, divorced from distractions, our mind is sufficiently quiet to be aware of what we are doing when we start to rise from a chair. In our habitual mode this is likely to involve a host of extraneous, unhelpful movements and tensions – pulling back our head, hollowing our back, tensing our shoulders and so on. So the first thing we're encouraged to do is to stop doing it. By consciously forestalling our habitual reaction, we can allow the relationship of our head and back to remain balanced and flexible. We remain in a condition of **release**, in which we are poised to choose how to engage ourselves most efficiently to achieve the desired result. The outcome is the continuous positive cycle of Fig 1.8, reinforcing both physical and psychological ease.

What emerges from this account is that the *AT* is first and foremost about *breaking the force of habit*. It is not intended as a method for replacing bad habits with good ones. Inasmuch as habits are unthinking, the *AT* shuns them altogether. In the words of the philosopher William James, who had a high regard for Alexander's work, "The only habit to cultivate is the habit of giving up habits". True awareness is thinking in the moment and not relying on habit. Only in this way can we approach any situation with a fresh and open mind. Greater awareness of our use brings with it the challenge of exploration and genuine discovery.

Awareness in the Water

How can this sense of discovery be applied to swimming? Most swimmers are locked into unthinking patterns of behaviour in the water. These range from swimming with the head pulled back regardless of the pain and strain it produces, to ploughing through the water for long periods in a mindless fashion. Such patterns often stem from fears or persistent misapprehensions which have never been properly articulated or questioned. They serve as a block to achieving a sense of true freedom in the water, and lead to feelings of boredom and apathy about swimming. Tackling these patterns at their root frees the spirit of exploration, which enlivens the whole process of swimming. Every stroke becomes an opportunity for discovery and self-exploration, expanding our horizon and opening up a new realm of possibility. Recognising the consistent interconnection between mental and physical habits, and becoming aware of mindless patterns, are the first steps towards acquiring the ability to approach the water without anxiety or strain.

Conventional swimming teaching rarely recognises how the force of habit gets in the way of learning. The assumption is that if learners are told or shown how to do something, they will be able to do it. The problem is that habits dictate our whole pattern of action. Although they can offer a short cut to building up our skills, they can also impede the optimum development of those skills. Once they have become fixed, they can be very hard to dislodge. These habits of both thought and action are observable in swimmers at all levels. Whether it's the beginner pulling back his head in response to water splashing in his face, or the Olympic swimmer developing an unexpected stroke fault in her effort to win a race, their problems can be traced to their inability to overcome an unthinking habit.

By its nature, the swimming environment is likely to present greater distractions than an *AT* teaching room. On top of external distractions, swimmers have to contend with their private feelings about being lightly-clad, getting wet, submerging their face in water, swimming in public, and numerous other more-or-less unexpressed anxieties. It's a tremendous challenge to retain one's awareness under such conditions! Anxiety often has the apparent effect of heightening one's awareness, because it intensifies certain sensations. You will have noticed how under intimidating conditions lights can seem brighter, distances larger, and noises louder. In fact, these very responses take your awareness away from your self and your relationship to the immediate surroundings. What's required under these circumstances is to quieten your mind. The *AT* encourages this by directing your attention, in the first instance, to the fundamental aspect of your use – the relationship between your head, neck and back, the **primary control**.

There is another side to the coin: water can be an extremely liberating, reflective, and sensual medium for exploration. It has exciting and unusual properties. For instance, buoyancy allows us to get as close to weightlessness as we are likely to experience without travelling into space. Liquidity offers the possibility of uniquely pleasurable sensations. Being submerged in water has well-known calming and uplifting effects. Water challenges us to discover how to use our whole body to manoeuvre through it successfully. It magnifies the effects of good and bad use. For example, the effect of pulling the head backwards and down can be more noticeable in the water than outside: it causes the lower body to sink down, creating greater resistance to our attempts at propulsion. Factors of this kind can waken in us a greater awareness of our immediate experience.

Even when we are sufficiently used to our surroundings for them not to be a distraction, another familiar habitual tendency comes into play: the desire to make active efforts to achieve our ends. This is related to the whole issue of **end-gaining** outlined above, and will be discussed in greater detail in the following chapter. At this stage it should be reiterated that the first steps to awareness involve precisely the opposite of making active efforts. Before any benefit can arise, first you have to stop and do nothing. Just by dropping the habit of being more active than you need, you allow yourself to remain constantly aware of your habitual reactions and your **use.**

This applies to each and every stage of your approach to the water: the efforts you make when changing into swim-wear, when walking to the pool, when getting into the water, when submerging your face, when performing a stroke. When it comes to acquiring new skills, swimmers of all levels are inclined to apply excessive effort. But as the case studies in this chapter show, even the first step in swimming – learning to float – is not something you actually *do.* In fact, trying to hold yourself up in the water has exactly the opposite effect. What one must learn is how to let go and allow the water to support the body. Being constantly on guard and learning to stop is the way to unlearn this habit. As the unnecessary obstacles posed by your efforts are stripped away, a virtuous cycle arises in which natural and effective water skills are allowed to emerge and flourish (see Fig 1.10). These bring about the quiet confidence that allows you to maintain awareness and enjoy the experience of being in the water.

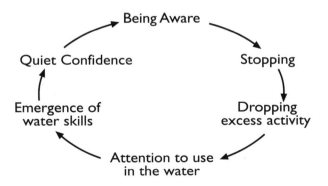

Fig 1.10

Case Study IA: Oliver – Learning to Float

At 30, Oliver was convinced that he had a fundamental problem with the water. Tall, thin, heavy-boned and muscular, he contended that he was simply unable to float. He imagined himself as a solid pole, prone to sink in the water like a stone. As a result, he would not get into the water without creating a great deal of movement with his arms and legs in order to try to keep himself afloat, and resolutely kept his head above the water surface to ensure that he could breathe. The result of his efforts was that he would rapidly become tired and breathless. The rigid position of his head above the water added to the natural tendency of his hips to sink under the weight of his long legs, and led to discomfort and neck-strain after just a short session in the water.

He was initially dubious when it was suggested that he would only float if he did less to prevent it. Although he understood that the air present in the body and lungs could be used to provide buoyancy for the whole body, he had never experienced floating because he had never allowed himself to lie still in the water and experience the sense of his torso lengthening and widening. He was first persuaded to release his head into the water, so that the new orientation of his upper body might allow his chest and lungs to act as a natural buoy. Although he initially sank below the surface, he found that if he did nothing his upper body eventually floated upwards, allowing him to breathe simply by lifting his head. After a few lessons of just gliding without moving his arms and legs, he became aware of how he had been locking the well-developed muscles of his torso in an effort to hold himself up in the water. The less he actually tried to do, the more he could allow his upper body to assert its natural buoyancy.

Primary Control in the Water

As outlined above, a central concept of the *AT* is the primary control – the relationship between the head, neck and back in governing the overall use and functioning of the body. The relation of the head to the rest of the body is crucial to establishing poise and freedom of movement, because of its effect on the contraction and extension of the spinal column, the muscles of the neck and upper body – and through these on the rib-cage, breathing apparatus, and our whole musculo-skeletal structure. This relationship is truly dynamic: virtually every movement we make involves a change in it. At the heart of the *AT* is the concept that we can replace unconscious alterations to this balance, which work to our detriment, with conscious adjustments that work in favour of helping our body to function efficiently. The habitual response of pulling the head backwards and down is prevented by conscious decision. In its place, at every opportunity, we can discover a more natural and healthy response which allows for lengthening and widening throughout the body.

In the water, even a small re-alignment of the head and neck can have a dramatic effect on the balance and orientation of the body. Because of the body's horizontal position, the head acts as an important counterweight and agent of balance. In particular, when the head is pulled back in the prone strokes, it dramatically alters the balance of the whole body so that the hips immediately begin to sink (when swimming on the back, the same effect results from pushing the head forward).

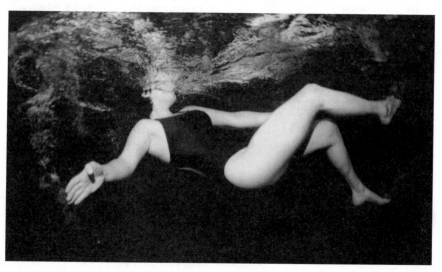

Fig 1.11
*As the head lifts, the hips sink – whether swimming
on front or back.*

Swimmers who concentrate on propulsion through the water commonly focus on their arms and legs, and pay insufficient attention to the use of the whole body. As a result the majority of swimmers have little awareness of how their head is behaving relative to the rest of their body when they swim. Standard swimming manuals lay stress on body position as a key element in swimming technique. However, this can imply an over-rigid positioning of one's head relative to the rest of the body, which militates against good use in the water. It's not body *position*, but a

forward-and-upward *direction* and a dynamic balance of one's whole physical structure that are all-important. The importance of the primary control for bringing this about will be explored in a later chapter on **Leading with the Head: Orientation & Balance**.

Case Study 1B: Ruth – Learning the Breast Stroke

Ruth enjoyed swimming but encountered the common problem of being unable to co-ordinate the breast stroke in a satisfactory way. However rapidly she moved her arms and legs she could not achieve steady progress through the water. She found the experience difficult and tiring, taking up to 15 strokes to swim across the width of the pool. A former dancer, her problems with co-ordination were exclusive to the water, and she sought instruction to help her with her difficulties. Her belief that she needed to learn to move the right way was only half the story.

When she practised the stroke under supervision, she was shown how the immediate effect of action by the arms and legs was to make the body slow down. She became aware how each time she pulled up her knees her body momentarily stopped gliding steadily through the water. It became clear that the only time she actually moved for any length of time through the water was after her powerful leg-kick, when simply doing nothing allowed her body to glide forward, relaxed and fully extended. By taking full advantage of this, she discovered that the new orientation of her body allowed her more time to think and explore the optimum co-ordination of her arms and legs. In doing so, she found herself traversing the width easily with only four kicks.

Conclusion

A man is but the product of his thoughts: what he thinks, he becomes.

Mahatma Gandhi

This chapter has introduced the range of different concepts used in the Alexander Technique: the unity of the self, psychophysical awareness, habit and inhibition, the unreliability of sensation, use and misuse, and the primary control. It has outlined how these concepts can be applied and developed in the water, to establish a basis for effective swimming and to enhance the quality of the experience. While the emphasis of the *AT* in practice can appear to be on purely physical aspects of activity, the intimate connection of mental and physical is considered to be present at every level of action. Creating a more balanced head-neck-back relationship helps us to *think* more freely about our use, while increased attention to use brings about greater *physical* ease. In practising the *AT,* cause and effect are linked in a circular process of continuous positive feedback.

The mental space created by increased physical ease allows us to expand our attention and explore our *self* constructively in all types and aspects of activity. The development of awareness through the *AT* is invaluable as a preparation for changing our patterns of behaviour and developing new skills. Because of the unique and unusual properties of water, the specific application of the *AT* to an aquatic environment opens up new possibilities for experience and exploration. Most philosophies concur that we only experience life to the full when we live totally in the present. Not only does practice of the Technique offer indications about how we might think constructively about swimming, but the lessons of awareness in the water expand our potential to understand the way we use ourselves from moment to moment outside the water.

The remainder of this book looks in detail at the aspects of the *AT* outlined in this chapter, and explores how they can be effectively integrated with the key elements of swimming. In the course of our exploration it should become clear how both the *AT* and the art of swimming have a wider significance than might at first be imagined. Both invite philosophical reflections that are grounded in human experience: ideas of change, flow, balance and harmony. Together they open up a new vista of possibilities for growth and self-development.

2. Fitness Can Damage Your Health!

Know Thyself. Nothing in Excess.   Ancient Greek wisdom

Know your limits...then BREAK THEM!   Printed on a sports T-shirt

High-speed travel and electronic media dominate our lives and continue to proliferate into the 21st century. They have already led to a huge increase in sedentary occupations and diminished our active physical involvement with the environment. Nowadays we no longer need to use our bodies in the way our ancestors did. Despite technology's undoubted potential for liberation, the wonders of the hi-tech age are an incitement to physical and mental laziness. In the wake of explosive technological growth, the lives of individuals are progressively alienated from activities which require a balanced use of the whole self. Our way of living and working encourages physical inactivity. As a result, the lack of adequate, regular exercise has become a cause of disease and ill-health in modern industrialised societies. Technology so permeates our lives that we have come to associate even the idea of fitness with rows of electronic machines. Even when we exercise we want machines to do the work for us.

Despite the constant pressure to "get fit", most people in modern industrial societies still run a mile to avoid regular exercise! Some can't be bothered: when seized by the urge to take exercise... they lie down until it passes. Others actively resist exercise because it feels such a strenuous, uncomfortable, and tedious way of spending time. They are apparently oblivious to the message that it can make a vital contribution to their health and quality of life. There is clear evidence that regular aerobic exercise reduces the risks of coronaries, strokes and heart disease. It enhances

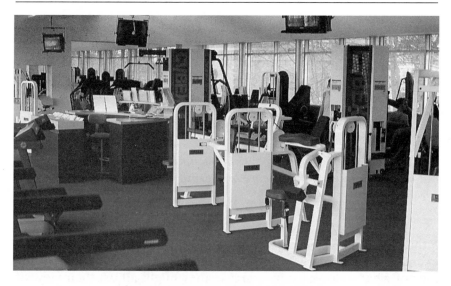

Fig 2.1 *Exercise in a hi-tech age.*

cardiovascular efficiency and encourages fuller breathing, helping
to regulate blood pressure and reduce stress. Better breathing and
circulation boost mental functioning, and hormones such as the
endorphins which are stimulated by vigorous activity have a
revitalising effect on our system. As a result, exercise can bring
about a noticeable increase in energy and vitality. *So long as it is
performed in an intelligent manner*, exercise undoubtedly has the
potential to promote health and longevity, and bring about a sense
of greater well-being.

But how intelligent are we about exercising? Surrounded by
noise and haste, we tend to match extreme situations with extreme
responses. When we feel we have gone wrong, we so often seek to
redress the balance with something equally wrong! In the face of ill-
health caused by inactive life-styles, our characteristically
unbalanced response is to pursue a dubious ideal of fitness. So on
the one hand there is unhealthy inactivity, on the other all the
absurdities of the latest fitness boom. Fitness is the fashion. The
desire to appear fit has resulted in a growing incidence of anorexic
emaciation, spinal injuries, steroid abuse, and strained muscles.
Commercial organisations and the media continually reinforce the
message: *thou shalt be fit*. As a result, more people than ever go
jogging, cycle, work out, swim, and indulge in other forms of
exercise with fitness as the stated goal. They express feelings of guilt
and shame for not exercising enough. They launch into activity,

adopting at second-hand a thinly considered approach which denies a whole spectrum of possibilities for balanced change. Their response exemplifies the words of F.M. Alexander: the opposite of wrong is wrong.

Fitness and Health

Health is a state of complete physical, mental and social well-being, and not merely the absence of disease or infirmity.

The World Health Organization

Fitness is usually the explicit goal of people who pursue regular exercise. But do they know what they mean by it? With a clearer idea of what to look for in exercise, they might adjust their view of how to do it. So what is a healthy approach to fitness? While exercise brings indisputable benefits, fitness is not synonymous with health. We all know that some people can appear very "fit" but be quite *un*healthy.

Take a moment to ask yourself what "fitness" means to you. A better understanding of what you mean by "fitness" throws light on how and why you pursue it. By learning to make the best use of your time and energy, you ultimately stand to enhance immeasurably the value of the exercise you take - and of any activity you choose to engage in.

When we do strenuous, repetitive exercise for the sake of fitness, are we aware of what is really happening to our bodies? We are encouraged to think that a trim, muscular or athletic image should make us more attractive (or at least feel more attractive). But insight into what we do to ourselves when we exercise can provide the catalyst for radical change in our approach to the whole question of fitness and health. The value of a fitness regime which is frankly boring, painful, and may result in chronic injury is, to say the least, questionable! A good reason for staying fit, however, is to be able to take vigorous activity for a reasonable period of time without feeling unduly breathless, strained or exhausted. This has clear benefits for all sorts of activities we encounter in daily life - climbing stairs, running for a bus, carrying heavy objects. Cardiovascular fitness obtained through regular aerobic exercise

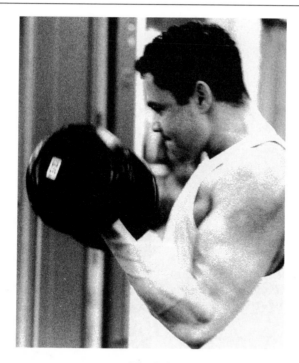

Fig 2.2
The weight-trainer's determination shows in every muscle.

certainly increases the chances of longevity. But long life is only
something to be desired if we remain in a condition to enjoy it:
staying fit through regular exercise can help enhance the quality of
our lives by sharpening our faculties and allowing us to enjoy a
wide range of physical and intellectual activities into old age. All
these are valid enough reasons for wanting to undertake a balanced
regime of physical activity.

As well as forming a clearer idea of our aims in taking exercise,
before embarking on a fitness routine we are customarily
encouraged to be aware of our overall physical condition. But such
an awareness, as we discussed in the previous chapter, exists on
different levels. You may not, for instance, suffer from a specific
medical condition or physical deficiency which prevents you
exercising. Are you sufficiently in touch with yourself, even when
simply sitting or standing, to know that the way you choose to
exercise will bring the desired benefits? Can you be sure that it
doesn't pose risks to your health in ways that you overlook?

Take breathing, for instance. It's essential to good health and a
key aspect of the art of swimming. Ineffective breathing can

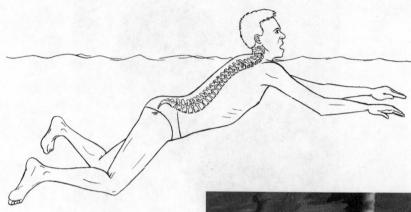

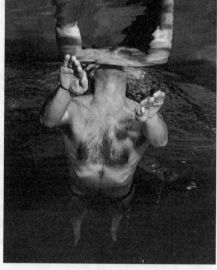

Fig 2.3
*Two views of a swimmer with
the head pulled back, showing
how stress can occur.*

significantly reduce, if not nullify, the positive effects of exercise. Are you aware of how you breathe, and how your breathing changes during different types of activity? Or take the desire to look good. The single-minded pursuit of muscular strength and a "good figure" can have particularly unwelcome side-effects. Are you sure that straining to extend your muscles is not placing dangerous pressure on your joints and tendons? Are you aware that excessive muscle build-up can reduce your flexibility, lead to rheumatic problems, and cause increasing discomfort as time goes on? [1]

---

[1] A major Finnish study (reported in the British Medical Journal 1994) showed conclusively that top athletes are at significantly higher risk of premature disease of the weight-bearing joints.

One reason why swimming is such a popular fitness pursuit is because it is thought to promote health and well-being without such injurious side-effects. It is recommended by doctors as a remedial activity for chronic conditions, and is considered suitable for all ages and physical types. The advantages of swimming over other forms of exercise are often cited as follows:

1. Properties of buoyancy and density allow vigorous exercise in water with a low risk of injury.
2. Swimming requires the use of the whole body in a balanced and integrated manner.
3. Swimming is safer because it encourages a steady, rather than rapid increase in cardiovascular activity.[2]
4. Water itself has relaxing and therapeutic properties which help make swimming enjoyable as well as beneficial.

The pursuit of fitness aims to address three areas of physical capability: strength, stamina, and suppleness. When charts are provided showing how different types of exercise rate in these respects, swimming usually heads the list. At least, swimming emerges as the exercise which supplies the best overall balance of conventional fitness requirements, as illustrated by the chart below.

	Strength	Stamina	Suppleness
Swimming:	● ● ●	● ● ● ●	● ● ● ●
Cycling:	● ● ●	● ● ● ●	● ●
Weight training:	● ● ● ●	● ●	●
Yoga:	●	● ●	● ● ● ●
Jogging:	● ●	● ● ●	● ●

What such a chart doesn't indicate is the level of risk presented by the different forms of exercise – their potential for pain, strain and injury. In fact, any form of exercise, if taken to extremes, can have detrimental effects on health both in the short term and the long term. If we exercise without sufficient forethought or attention, there's always some degree of risk. The growing incidence of sports-related injuries has led to increasing recognition of the dangers of highly strenuous types of exercise,

---

[2] For this reason swimming is often particularly recommended for people with heart problems. This is not to deny the importance of a warm-up period for all forms of exercise and vigorous activity, if one is to avoid the risk of injury to muscles and joints.

such as those involving weights. Swimming is put in a category of low-impact exercises which are supposedly exempt from such risks. But there's a way in which even low-impact exercise may cause harm: if the effect of one's actions is to compound pre-existing strains, tension and rigidity. This is rarely given sufficient consideration, and here the Alexander Technique has an important insight to offer. "Fitness" becomes a dubious pursuit for those whose system is out of balance: unless they pay attention to their *use*, virtually any kind of exercise can cause harm or discomfort, and will be of limited benefit.

It's sometimes claimed that exercise needs to hurt to have any effect – the "no pain, no gain" syndrome. Not only is this suspiciously masochistic, but it creates a double-bind: the attempt simultaneously to inflict pain on oneself and to be indifferent to it. How confusing! If we learn to enjoy the sensation of pain by deliberately straining to the point of excess, the body's natural mechanisms, which normally seek to make us aware of discomfort so that we can take measures to reduce it, are thrown into turmoil. So, by pursuing fitness in this way, we set up a conflict of feelings which ends up with us actively blocking our awareness.

Nor do we help ourselves when the exercise environment itself is not conducive to sensitivity. The heavy beat of music in group aerobic sessions, the hubbub of the gym bustling with noise and activity, and a host of other distractions can overload the senses and divert our attention from our immediate experience. Equally distracting is the internal clamour – the desire to look good, to show off, to keep up with others, to conceal one's figure, to avoid the tedium of exercise by letting the mind wander. The fact that exercise, and especially swimming, often takes place in a public environment makes such distractions hard to avoid, particularly when they are not recognised as potentially harmful and handled accordingly. One of the most unhelpful internal pressures is the urge to compete in the water, which is so common and widely accepted that it merits further consideration here.

Learning to Swim: The Competitive Model

The public image of swimming is shaped by what we see and read on our television screens and in the media. These are mainly competitive events in which the sole criterion of success in the water is *speed*. In competitive swimming, as in every other sport, records are being broken all the time. Sports science has revolutionised the way that top athletes train and swim, and human velocity in the water has increased in leaps and bounds.[3] This is part and parcel of the modern world's obsession with speed. There are no Gold Medals for running gracefully or swimming freestyle in a supremely elegant way! The emphasis on speed dominates the way that we think about swimming. It affects our view of swimming at all levels, as swimmers seek to emulate the style and achievement of champions.

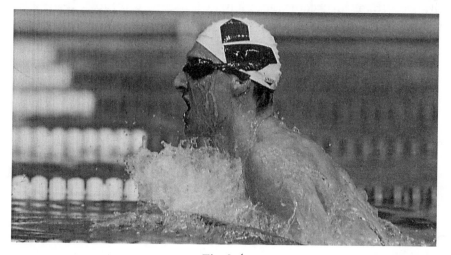

Fig 2.4

But is it hard to fathom that this attitude – speed at any cost – may be inappropriate for the *average* swimmer? Given that we haven't developed the physical capacities that allow top athletes to exploit their natural talents under extreme conditions, not only is focusing on speed more likely to result in strain, but it's bound to distort our understanding of how to swim more enjoyably and

---

[3] The record for swimming 100 metres is a telling example. In 1936 Johnny Weissmuller stunned the world when he swam 100 metres in under a minute. The current world record is under 50 seconds: Weissmuller would be trailing today's champion by *over a quarter of the length* of a 50-metre Olympic-size pool!

effectively at our own level. We unconsciously absorb, for instance, skilfully captured images of Olympic breast-stroke sprinters pulling themselves high out of the water with every stroke. This over-exertion may be one way of helping the contestant swim the breast stroke faster in his or her single-minded race to the end of the pool. But the cost of doing so is tremendous pressure on the lower back and torso. How can this help *you* to attain a healthier and happier experience of swimming? It's far likelier to cause discomfort and even pain.

Fitness enthusiasts often treat swimming as just another form of physical training. Reluctant exercisers also take the opportunity to delude themselves that swimming is an easy route to fitness: given swimming's well-known benefits, the occasional dip, the routine 20 lengths, is enough to assuage their guilt about lack of serious exercise. Even those who ostensibly go swimming "for fun" can slip into the habit of treating it solely as a means to fitness. Ironically,

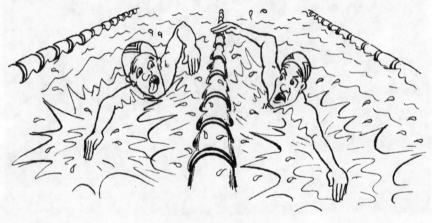

Fig 2.5 *Lane Rage.*

they may choose the water in the first place because they appreciate that swimming offers unique varieties of pleasure which land-based activities cannot. But nine times out of ten, their attitude to what they *should* do in the water circumscribes their ability to enjoy the very qualities that make swimming such a distinctive recreational activity.

In particular, we often observe people who clearly think of themselves as good swimmers totally intent on covering a stretch of water in the fastest possible time. The water becomes an assault-course for them as they thrash up and down with unflinching determination but no sense of exploration. They may as well not be in water at all, given that they're using it merely as another piece of gym apparatus against which to push and heave. Exercising in the water for the sake of fitness all too often takes on the character of a duty rather than a pleasure.

These approaches all exemplify a *lack of attention to the moment-by-moment experience*, which frequently has its origin in our early experience. Such inattention is often the unhappy result of learning to swim in a way which overemphasises competitive goals. Most young children see the water as a "favourite place" – a space to play, have fun, and experience sensations that are exciting and different. Fear of water is not innate. It usually arises out of negative attitudes or experiences in early youth (these are discussed in greater detail in Chapter 3). Other reasons for many adults' reluctance to swim may similarly be due to pressures experienced at an early age. All too often, children who demonstrate a marked degree of ability in the water are urged by over-ambitious teachers or parents to "get serious about swimming". This can mean embarking on a strenuous training programme from a very early age. It's questionable how much a 10-year-old can benefit from being pushed to the limit of his or her physical ability for up to four hours a day! Inevitably, the sense of fun will be subordinated to a desire to swim faster or further than the next child. Although competition can be useful for developing skills to a high level, it can also be counterproductive: it implies that activity is not an end in itself but a means to some external reward. Official swimming-teaching organisations encourage this by promoting an incentive-based model of achievement – badges, medals and awards – which unfortunately allows little room for initiative or creativity in the water. While such incentives work for some, for others they interfere with the discovery of personal enjoyment in swimming, and turn it into a sport in which artificial, pre-defined ends hold more allure than the activity itself.

The competitive approach can become so ingrained that it's very hard to shake off in later life. Teenagers and adults often retain competitive attitudes even when they are no longer in a competitive setting. Although their skills may easily be adequate for them to explore the water's qualities creatively and in a non-competitive way, they are stuck with a mind-set of which they are only vaguely aware. Former competition swimmers are often completely turned off any desire to swim once their competitive stint comes to an end. If they do venture into the water, it's without any sense of fun. In their mind's ear they hear the brusque commands or nagging criticism of coach or parent. They enter a pool with the fixed intention of completing their lengths in a given time, and adopt a competitive and even aggressive stance towards others whom they encounter alongside.

The competitive attitude also produces a definite resistance to the idea of change. Any change – especially a substantial change of approach – requires a period of adjustment in which a sense of disorientation is likely to arise. Because competition swimmers have developed vested interests in speed, change is particularly hard for them. They are afraid they will be taking a backward step if they drop their focus on speed. But if they allow themselves to do so, they can begin to awaken to a whole new realm of enjoyment. For practised competitors, discovering an art of swimming which removes the emphasis on goals can arouse a new and unfamiliar pleasure in the creative exploration of their hard-won aquatic skills.

Case Study 2A: Jason – Learning to Win Again

Jason was referred to the Alexander Technique with back problems connected to years of competitive swimming. A lover of water from youth, he had been trained to plough up and down the pool for hours at a time to increase his speed and endurance. The competitive environment gave him little room to think about the way he was swimming. In his effort to reach the end of the pool first he would constantly look ahead by pulling his head back, which had the effect of stiffening his neck and shortening his stature even while he sought to redouble his efforts to reach the far side sooner. The tremendous muscular effort needed to move through the water in this way put further pressure on his lungs and spine, resulting in chest pains and a chronic condition resembling whiplash.

As a result he gave up competitive swimming, but whenever he entered the water he found it hard to resist his competitive training and would swim at full stretch regardless of the consequences. At a reunion of his swimming team he noted the general consensus: the strain of competitive swimming had put most of them off swimming altogether! Learning the Alexander Technique encouraged Jason to rethink his approach to swimming. He realised that his back problems stemmed from his attitude, that of an extreme end-gainer. He retrained himself to swim without trying to come first all the time by exerting excessive muscular effort. The main fruit of his change of attitude was, for him, that for the first time since he was a young child he remembered how it felt to *love* swimming.

An End to End-Gaining

Modern man thinks he loses something – time – when he does not do things quickly; yet he does not know what to do with the time he gains – except kill it.

Erich Fromm

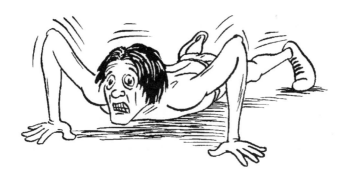

Fig 2.6
"17, 18, 19, 20 ..."

The fitness enthusiast and the competition swimmer as described above demonstrate instances of the attitude which in the *AT* is termed "end-gaining". Focussing on the attainment of a distant goal prevents us from paying sufficient attention to the processes involved. This both hinders our ability to attain the desired end and does nothing to enhance the quality of our experience. Exercises that are performed in sets, such as weight-lifting, sit-ups and press-ups, are particularly conducive to an end-gaining mind-set. If we are concerned about getting to the end of the set of exercises without collapsing, we are less likely to be concerned with and pay due attention to the way we are using or *mis*using our body.

We have seen how the pursuit of fitness itself offers a prime example of the drawbacks of end-gaining. Although modern culture advocates strenuous exercise to improve our mental and physical condition, there's not enough critical debate about the benefits it is alleged to provide. In fact, even a little more sensitivity to the working of our organism as a whole enables us to notice how fitness regimes can work against our natural balance. Exercise programmes tend to reinforce bad habits and misuse, and the tendency to stiffen the neck and pull the head back is exaggerated as the speed of movement or the effort required increases.

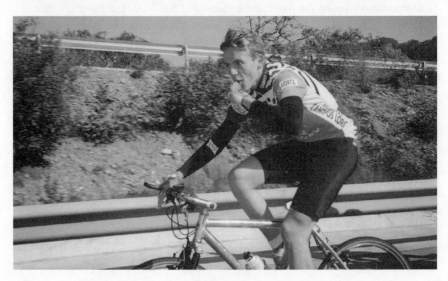

Fig 2.7
The cyclist: misuse is exaggerated as speed increases.

Some routines deliberately treat us like machines whose component parts can be worked on and built up in isolation from the functioning of the whole. Mechanical activity which isolates individual muscle groups in this way is prone to ignore the integrated nature of a healthily functioning musculo-skeletal system. It can result in our developing some areas of our body disproportionately, thereby reducing our overall flexibility and impeding the smooth functioning of the joints. Furthermore, such routines smother our sensitivity. The body's signals of misuse, such as persistent aches and pains, are ignored in the drive to improve our "form". It's not surprising that the incidence of exercise-related injury grows year by year, and that sports-related therapies – virtually unknown a decade ago to all except professional athletes – have become a regular feature of the modern fitness scene.

Sports medicine has identified a wide range of specific injuries sustained by competitive swimmers, such as a form of tendonitis referred to as "swimmer's shoulder", and disabling pain caused by the erosion of cartilage around the knee ("breast-stroker's knee"). Much more common is the unpleasant experience of cramp in the water. This is most often due to the inadvertent over-extension of less-used muscles in the legs and torso. Although swimming is alleged to be innocuous, it clearly presents risks if pursued in an unconsidered way. It's important to be aware of the potential hazards, and to know how strain and injury can occur despite the fact that the water acts as a cushion against 'high-impact' injury.

The support offered to the body by water, with its dual property of both yielding to and resisting our actions, certainly offers us the opportunity to increase strength and stamina while moving more freely and fluidly than is possible on land. Swimmers intent on achieving a goal of fitness rarely appreciate these advantages to the full: their ease and enjoyment are impeded by the sheer effort of trying to swim a given distance in a set time, in an inflexible way. If their system is already out of balance, even the advantages of buoyancy in reducing the requirement for effort are not realised: the unhealthy imbalance is merely reinforced. Excessive effort and poor technique can actually do more harm than good. Swimming awkwardly can reactivate old injuries, aggravate disorders, and result in neck, shoulder and back pain.

End-gaining thus serves little purpose apart from providing a distraction to performing the activity in hand. Those who swim with the overriding intention in their minds to get fit, strengthen their muscles, or lose weight – typical examples of end-gaining approaches – usually have fixed ideas of *what* they should do to achieve their aims. Little thought is given to the way they move through the water; attention is switched off and automatic habits take over. This tendency can be a major obstacle to learning to be free and feeling at home in the water. Even though the buoyancy of water in principle reduces the need for effort and can accordingly have a positive effect on our use, in practice few swimmers have sufficient awareness of their use to develop a style for themselves that exploits this advantage to the full. So *don't try*! Instead, if you have specific goals, be aware of how focussing on the end can actually hinder you from attending to the most effective way of achieving the desired result. You can take the first step to a new and healthier way of swimming simply by *reconsidering your motivation for being in the water.*

The method proposed by the *AT* of overcoming the drawbacks of end-gaining in practice is to learn to pay attention to the intermediate steps (this was called by F.M. Alexander "attending to the means-whereby"). By eliminating the unnecessary pressure caused by trying to attain a particular end, one can become more aware of the moment and thereby achieve greater command over one's thoughts and actions – in other words, greater control of the whole self. The removal of an automatic end-gaining response makes it possible for a more mindful attitude to emerge, resulting in more effective learning.

A mechanical routine which smothers awareness by setting artificial goals is apt to suppress unarticulated anxieties in the process. This is another way in which the blind pursuit of fitness goals can be dangerously counterproductive: anxieties (discussed in more detail in Chapter 3) remain obscured to their owner, only to emerge in awkward symptoms such as stroke defects and strained breathing. In the urge to achieve a stronger or faster stroke, swimmers develop awkward movements without realising it. In addition, problems of style which swimmers already display may be exacerbated as they plough on unawares. It's often only by revealing fears clearly and explicitly that they can be systematically addressed and overcome.

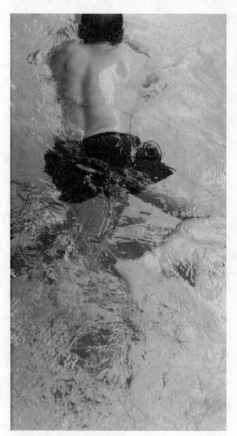

For example, the involuntary twisting round of one leg in the breast stroke (known as the 'screw-kick') sets up a negative chain of movements throughout the body. This places uneven pressure on the hips, lower back, and ultimately the entire spinal column. The tendency is very hard to eradicate, and can only be effectively countered by careful attention and the mindful practice, lying on both front and back, of moving both legs symmetrically. Swimmers who remain excessively focussed on fitness goals are unlikely to be able to correct this often deeply ingrained and potentially harmful stroke defect.

Fig 2.8
A "screw-kick" affects the whole body, not just the legs.

Case Study 2B: Helen – Getting Fit to Swim

Helen booked a beginner's course with the avowed intention of learning to swim in order to get fit and lose weight. She had a preconceived idea that the way to achieve this was to employ maximum effort, both as a way of staying afloat and of burning calories. She resisted all suggestions to let go and apply less effort, with the result that after several sessions she was still thrashing about energetically, but unable to stay afloat or swim for any distance. After several more sessions it became apparent that one reason for her excessive effort was a long-held anxiety about appearing to be lazy. This unproductive thought had led to constant overdoing in her life generally.

When she started thinking about *not doing* she understood that she would only learn to swim if first she learned to float. This involved letting go of her notions about getting fit or actively doing anything to remain afloat. Setting aside her determination to derive immediate benefit from water exercise, she found that she could allow herself to experience the sensation of being supported by the water. She soon learned to float with ease, and was able to develop a relaxed swimming style which allowed her to swim with pleasure more often and for longer periods at a time. Without trying hard she became noticeably fitter, and both her poise and body tone improved.

The Alexander Technique & Fitness

Unknown to ourselves, by unconscious mimicry, we set our pace by the machine; and the pace destroys us by destroying our most sensitive and delicate co-ordinations and controls.

F. M. Alexander

The Alexander Technique is sometimes perceived, even by some of those who teach it, as a system which precludes or even prohibits vigorous physical activity. But what mattered to Alexander is not so much what we do as how we do it. Nowadays we tend to lead our lives as if our head was not a part of our body. We imagine that our physical and cerebral functioning are quite distinct. As a result of the heavy emphasis on the mental aspects, we try to compensate by intermittently increasing the level of our physical activity, usually in the form of set periods of rapid exercise designed to work on the body alone. In this way, we believe, we can bring the two parts of our system, mental and physical, into some sort of balance. The sight of someone cycling hard on a gym cycle, head bowed, reading a newspaper, exemplifies this attitude. It is assumed that the activity

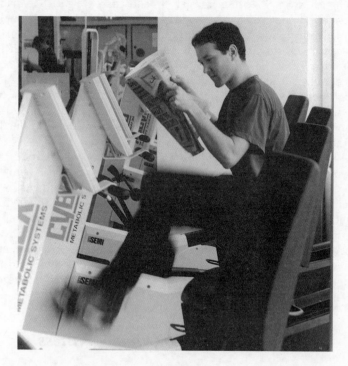

Fig 2.9
Keeping abreast of current affairs – but what about himself?

itself can benefit the body, even if the mind is not engaged in what we are doing.

But separating thinking from activity is fraught with danger. Mindless, repetitive action can be boring, pointless and potentially injurious. Such behaviour contrasts with what may be termed mindful activity, in which one's awareness unfolds from moment to moment – awareness both of oneself and the action in hand. In this mode, not only is one less liable to harm oneself through straining inadvertently, but the attention to the moment gives our actions a different quality of energy, productive of a range of positive effects both of a psychological and physical nature.

The concept of fitness itself, as we have suggested, is open to different interpretations, but it is usually promoted as the improvement of physical capability in isolation from emotional and psychological well-being. The latter are considered irrelevant or secondary, and as a result the pursuit of fitness becomes largely divorced from the way we think, move, and in general use ourselves

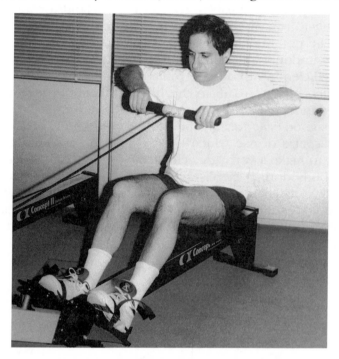

Fig 2.10
Mindful exercise: paying attention to the means-whereby.

in daily life. From an *AT* perspective, a more complete definition of fitness involves at least an appreciation of the overriding role of *use*, with its intimate relationship to good health and psychological well-being. F.M. Alexander was emphatic that bouts of strenuous exercise, practised in a mechanical fashion by people engaged in mainly sedentary occupations, could be harmful both psychologically and physically. "The body becomes the scene of a civil war", he wrote in *Man's Supreme Inheritance*, "in a state of perpetual re-adjustment to opposing conditions". In his view, exercise could not be treated in isolation from the way we use ourselves in our everyday lives, whether sitting, standing, walking, or lying down. From the broader perspective of the *AT*, unfitness and ill-health are primarily a consequence of misuse. Because every action we make contributes to or detracts from our level of health, the pursuit of fitness needs to be integrated into, rather than set apart from, the way we use ourselves in our day-to-day activities.

According to the *AT*, therefore, most exercise regimes are bound simply to reinforce bad habits. Someone who stands or walks badly is not likely to run or cycle any better: exercise will exaggerate the misuse. The potential benefits of a strong heart to an individual's health are undoubtedly reduced if other parts of the body are not working efficiently. Although aerobic fitness is important, it is only one aspect of the road to health and cannot be effectively developed independently of attention to the elements of use, such as *release*, good *orientation*, and healthy *breathing*. The awareness of these aspects of use which is developed by practice of the *AT* allows us to make a conscious choice about how we use our mind and our body during exercise – whether we "think in activity" or succumb to automatic habits. In this respect, fitness of mind and body are indissolubly connected. Being fit is not a matter of external physical fitness alone, but must include the ability to think and feel intelligently before, during, and after exercise. From an *AT*

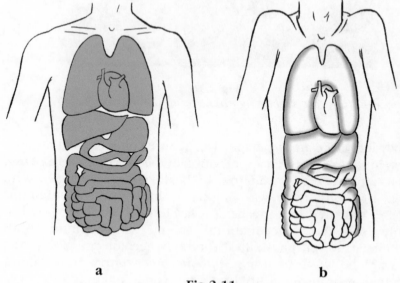

a   b

Fig 2.11
*For optimum functioning, internal organs should be free (a)
and not squashed together (b).*

perspective, any form of exercise should enhance, rather than detract from, the sensitivity and awareness of our use.

The *AT* approach thus creates something of a paradox, because it implies that you need to be fit *before* you can get fit! In other words, exercise cannot promote fitness if we are not already fit to exercise. The way Alexander proposed to overcome this Catch-22 was his emphasis on attending to the series of intermediate steps involve in any action, the means-whereby. This provides a method for both thought and activity to interact with one another in harmony, without either letting our thoughts outrun (or bypass) what happens in our body, or allowing our physical actions to blur our thinking.

The parallel condition, literally and symbolically, of our minds and bodies is shown in the previous illustration. When our bodies are cramped or restricted, the internal organs are forced up against each other, limiting their ability to function effectively. The heart, lungs, kidneys, intestines and so on can only function healthily if they are allowed to occupy their fair share of space. The congestion which results from misuse during strenuous activity interferes with their optimum operation. Equally, we need mental space if our thought process is to function at its optimum level. A quiet, attentive mind, free of irrelevant distractions, is necessary for us to perform vigorous exercise in a truly beneficial manner.

A relaxed and creative state of mind within a well-tuned body: this is the beginning and end of fitness, the optimum condition if we want to break free of ingrained attitudes, acquire new skills, and discover what true fitness can mean.

Steps to a New Approach

Here are a number of practical suggestions that can help to bring about a new sense of healthy exploration and enjoyment in the water. Characteristically, they act as reminders to ourselves to *let go* of habits that may have become quite automatic. Use them – singly, in groups, and all together – as promptings to self-exploration in the water. By letting go of the old habits, a better, more creative way of swimming can emerge.

Don't hold in your stomach or hunch your shoulders, before or on entering the water
It may be chilly, or others may be watching. But awareness of habits like this is important: the way you are before entering the water reflects and is bound to affect your disposition when you swim.

Avoid setting a target number of lengths and counting
20 lengths, 50 lengths, what does it prove? It only takes your mind off the actual swimming. Why give yourself irrelevant orders? Dropping this often unconsidered habit can be truly liberating.

Don't rush, but enjoy each stroke
A well-executed stroke is likely to have greater benefits for body-toning and aerobic build-up, as well as giving the space for mindful activity, than a flurry of movement made in the pursuit of a dubious fitness goal.

Don't hold your breath
This is often unconscious, in which case you need to make it conscious, so that you can learn to avoid breathlessness and hyperventilation. There is rarely any merit in deliberately holding your breath. It's likely to disturb your ability to think clearly about what you're doing.

Don't tense or hyperextend your body
This is one of the main causes of cramp. It detracts from both the elegance and efficiency of a stroke, and has detrimental effects on use both inside and outside the water.

Don't fight the water
You can only lose! Make the water your ally instead. Excessive effort is unnecessary and distracting, and in over-exerting yourself you fail to exploit the water's unique asset of buoyancy.

Don't compete
Why compare yourself with other swimmers at all? There is nothing to be gained, and much to be lost, by adopting other peoples' unconsidered goals and practices.

Pay attention to what you're doing without letting your mind wander
It's a good idea to think about painting when you paint, and cooking when you cook. That way you paint and cook better, and enjoy yourself more in the process. So why not pay attention to your swimming when you swim?

Experiment
You don't have to limit yourself to a set routine. Try something new and see what it feels like.

Smile!

It's surprising how few swimmers are aware of the extent to which they tense up their facial muscles. Smiling can draw your attention to this as well as helping to relax your face – an index of how relaxed the rest of your body is.

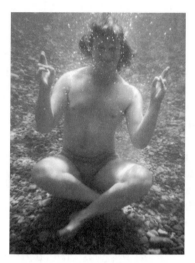

Fig 2.12

Conclusion

There is a Law of Reversed Effort. The harder we try with the conscious will to do something, the less we shall succeed. Proficiency and the results of proficiency come only to those who have learned the paradoxical art of doing and not doing.

Aldous Huxley

A common feature of the case histories in this chapter is the emphasis on trying to achieve, the sort of end-gaining that invariably accompanies the unthinking pursuit of fitness. We must be careful not to apply the same sort of trying to the task of learning a new approach, thus replacing one form of end-gaining with another! Alexander found that when pupils try to do the "right thing" they are inclined to apply the wrong sort of effort to the task, which actually prevents them from performing it efficiently. In his *Notes of Instruction* we read: "I don't want you to give a damn if you're right or not. Directly you don't care if you're right or not the impeding obstacle is gone." Swimmers who try to "do it the right way" create tensions which serve only to restrict their movements in the water. The anxiety aroused by trying to do the right thing is itself detrimental to awareness. The Alexander Technique shifts the emphasis away from trying to do the right thing to learning to prevent the wrong.

Learning to swim involves discovering how to control the body's natural buoyancy and make it work for you. As the body has a lower density than water, it will (almost always) float unless something is done to prevent it. Many adult beginners are reluctant to let the water support them, and may think that if they do nothing they will immediately sink to the bottom. Although there are individual physical differences which make it easier for some people to float than others, the main obstacle is the false notion that the body must actively be held up in the water. The idea of non-doing also applies in another way: swimming efficiently involves using the least effort to overcome resistance from the water. Applying too much effort increases friction and turbulence. Studies of Olympic swimmers have shown that the fastest swimmers are the ones who take the fewest strokes to cover the distance; what counts is not the amount of effort, but the appropriate use of effort.[4]

The principle of *non-doing* was crucial to Helen's recognition (see Case Study 2B on p.57) that thrashing about wouldn't help her learn to float, let alone swim. Non-doing is not the same as passivity or total inactivity: it's simply the result of a conscious decision not to respond in a habitual way. The Alexander Technique sets out to teach us how to consciously undo undesirable responses. A non-doing approach to swimming can work wonders both for the beginner and the more advanced swimmer: the less one does to hinder oneself, the easier it becomes to move through the water. This results in a truer approach to fitness which avoids the strain imposed by trying to attain inappropriate preconceived goals. A step-by-step, experimental approach allows swimmers to change unthinking or automatic responses both in and out of the water. Most of us act from unrecognised assumptions, about which we have a natural tendency to deceive both ourselves and others. Detecting some of the specific mental blocks which get in the way of swimming freely can be difficult. Some of the preliminary psychological obstacles, not usually given due consideration in the teaching of swimming, are discussed in the following chapter.

---

[4] This suggests a useful exercise in exploration: seeing how *few* strokes you need to take to swim a given distance without loss of momentum.

3. At Home in the Water

The only thing we have to fear is fear itself.　　Franklin D. Roosevelt

"I'm very brave generally", he went on in a low voice: "only today I happen to have a headache".

Lewis Carroll

What do we say when we observe a wonderful swimmer? "A fish in the water", "water-babies", "natural swimmers" – these are the sort of words we use. What separates such swimmers from those who are merely competent is clearly not just style or technique. They give the impression that there are no *psychological* barriers preventing them from interacting with the water in a complete and satisfying way. By contrast, one of the main obstacles in learning the art of swimming is the uncertainty that is so often felt about relating to the water. This ranges from persistent mild unease to attacks of sudden panic. The former constrains our freedom to explore the aquatic environment, and the latter can be as debilitating as full-scale aquaphobia. At either end of the spectrum, the thought of being surrounded by an alien medium results in feelings of psychological and physical discomfort. One can know how to swim, and even consider oneself a good swimmer, without feeling completely *at home* in the water.

Being at home in the water is a matter of trust. Trust in the water's ability to support the body without the need for us to hold ourselves up. Trust in our own ability to manoeuvre efficiently in a fluid medium. This trust comes about through understanding and familiarity. It needs to be cultivated and positively reinforced by our experience with water. Yet unfortunately our confidence is undermined by attitudes which we find hard to shake off. Recurring mistrust of the water and about our ability to negotiate it are self-fulfilling. But too often, such anxieties are swept under the carpet. Teachers and guidebooks don't deal adequately, if at all, with these issues. Swimmers themselves often deliberately trivialise and even deny them in the belief that they are best dealt with by being minimised or ignored. But the results of doing this can be far from trivial: it allows unhelpful reactions and feelings to be reinforced, and risks creating a vicious cycle of the kind we described in Chapter 1 (see Fig 1.8, p.32). To avoid such a scenario, anxieties of all kinds relating to swimming should always be dealt with sympathetically and appreciated for what they are.

Fear of water is not the same as respect for water. Even the strongest of swimmers ought to have a healthy respect for water and an awareness of its hazards. Powerful tides and currents – and in some waters, marine animals like sharks and jellyfish – can mean real danger for swimmers who don't heed warnings or take sensible precautions. It's foolish to take unnecessary risks or to be insufficiently prepared in any aquatic situation. Intelligence dictates that we acknowledge our limitations *vis-à-vis* the water and always take appropriate safety measures. Whilst accidents can occur as a result of misplaced over-confidence, fear itself is often the main factor that prevents us making an intelligent response. Fear can paralyse us both mentally and physically. It interferes with our breathing and our ability to control our movements, and stops us thinking clearly enough to manoeuvre our way out of danger. Over the longer term too, the dulling nature of unresolved anxieties and the cumulative effects of fear get in the way of intelligent learning and a creative response to our immediate situation.

Our Early Experience of Water

Child of Nature, learn to unlearn. Benjamin Disraeli

New-born babies have a natural affinity with water. We pass the first nine months or so after conception in a safe, controlled environment, entirely surrounded by water. Floating in the womb, our pre-natal experiences are pleasurable sensations of support, comfort and warmth. Perhaps it's this familiarity with the medium which gives babies a natural sense of being at home in the water: water-births are understandably becoming more popular. The ability to negotiate water without fear extends into the first few

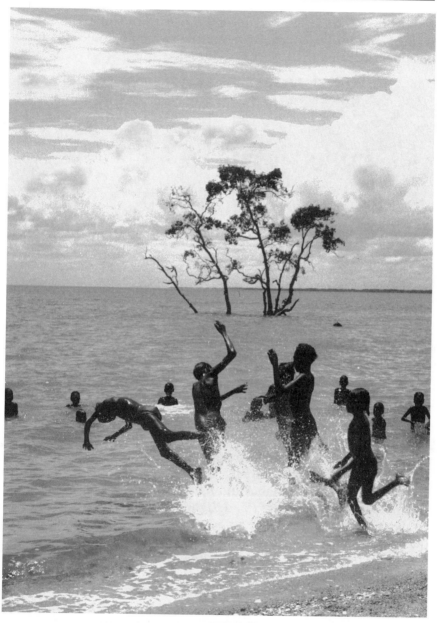

Fig 3.1

months of infancy. Swimming is classified as one of the *primitive reflexes*, along with, for example, the grasping reflex – the infant's automatic reaction to curl its hand around small objects. A baby immersed in water will move its limbs actively and automatically avoid breathing in: these reflexes keep it from sinking and from taking water into its lungs. However, the swimming reflex gradually disappears during the first year of life.

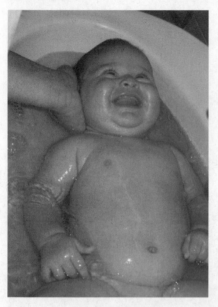
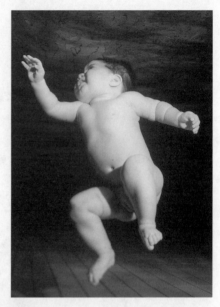

a   b
Fig 3.2
a) Supported by her mother's hand the baby enjoys the sensation of water.
b) A three-month old baby shows natural motor skills in the water.

When we observe small infants at bathtime we see how the water rarely presents a threat. As long as they feel secure and supported, it's a comfortable and pleasurable experience for them. Infant swimming classes are designed to build on this natural confidence before fears have an opportunity to set in. However, it's questionable whether formal swimming lessons at the infant stage are useful or desirable. There's a danger that both child and parent may acquire a false confidence in the infant's ability to cope in the water. It's unwise and surely inappropriate to expect very young children to be sufficiently safety-conscious on their own. Allowing them to play and have fun in water under adult supervision, rather than imposing on them such responsibility, is likely to be of more ultimate benefit.[1]

[1] In the wake of an increased incidence of infants drowning, the American Pediatric Association has expressed reservations about the wisdom of relying on infant swimming-classes to "waterproof" young children.

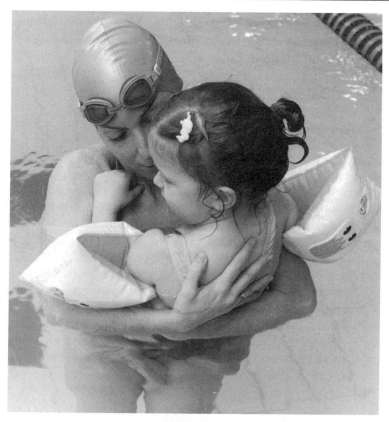

Fig 3.3
*Parents' attitudes vitally affect how a child
learns to relate to the water.*

The existence of a swimming reflex indicates that human beings have an *innate* ability – one that doesn't need to be taught – both to stay afloat and propel ourselves through the water. However, this can be *un*learned. Our attitude to the water is largely shaped during the psychologically critical period of our early years. Unfortunately, what *is* learned at this early stage is fear. This above all changes the quality of children's experience to one in which they no longer feel at home in the water. For most children, the early confidence about water is soon forgotten.

How does fear arise? The most common reason is that the child unconsciously notices and internalises the fears exhibited by parents or primary carers. When such individuals show anxiety about being in the water themselves, or make obvious their concern that the child is in danger, they unintentionally transmit their apprehensions to the child. Young children can be profoundly sensitive to such feelings when projected by a nervous parent or another person in their environment. The latters' sense of *not* being at home in water is strongly communicated. Other possible factors are subordinate to the overriding psychological impact of these messages. For example, the growing infant may recoil from the discomforts of being cold and wet, but this is only likely to develop into fear of water if the experience is associated with unhappy feelings of insecurity.

Many adults who express anxiety about swimming relate their fears to unhappy childhood experiences, most commonly one in which they felt that they were in danger of drowning. Such experiences can be so traumatic that they produce phobic reactions to water which can be very hard to overcome. They can result in the unreasonable conviction "I can't swim" – and more perniciously, in the excuse "I don't *want* to learn to swim because I don't like water". Not everyone, of course, has such an extreme reaction. Many people manage to swim despite their fears, but remarkably often a residual awkwardness or tension is apparent. We nearly all remain influenced by early experiences which act as a block to our progress in the water. Once we learn to appreciate their limiting effects, we can realise that a much fuller enjoyment of swimming may be gained by changing our whole approach to the water.

The Teaching of Fear

Most learning is not the result of instruction. It is rather the result of unhampered participation in a meaningful setting.
                                                                Ivan Illich

Fear is all around us. We go through life being afraid – of people, events, death, the unknown, ourselves, and of fear itself. One effect of fear is that it stops us reaching our full potential by getting in the way of our acquiring new knowledge and skills. This can result from those around us, even if they mean well, themselves being afraid of our growing, changing, and discovering our potential as individuals. Their fear on our behalf reflects their own fear of change. Life, however, is a constant process of change. While change can make us feel vulnerable, the alternative to embracing it is to live in a narrower world, surrounded by walls of fear and

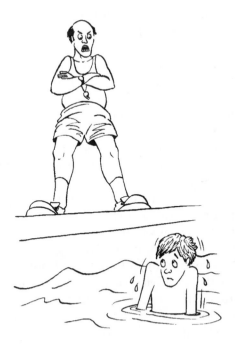

Fig 3.4
No false moves! Unfortunately, still a familiar scenario.

uncertainty. As this image suggests, by attempting to reject change we become restricted both in our bodies and our thinking. Fear disempowers us, making discovery of the *new* less appealing than repetition of the *known*. Whilst we may thus acquire a superficial sense of security, ultimately it leads to further insecurity – the consequence of stagnation and inflexibility. It stops us from thinking creatively, both in what we're doing and about how we want to experience our lives. We restrict ourselves through fear of humiliation, ignorance, solitude, society, pain, disease, or dying. And confusingly, sometimes through fear of growth, success, freedom, even love! At least we need to understand more clearly what we're afraid of if we wish to overcome the fear and move forward.

Systems of education and social and parental pressures insidiously encourage the development of fear. Trying to do something "right" – that is, in a way pleasing to those in authority – is the flip side of the fear of making mistakes. F.M. Alexander noted "If you could stop the tremendous effort of trying to be right, you might actually be able to achieve your desired end!" Making mistakes is an inevitable – and useful – part of the learning process. When we learn to speak a foreign language, we can't be concerned with speaking it correctly all the time or we are likely to remain tongue-tied. *If you recognise that you are doing something wrong, don't be annoyed with yourself: on the contrary, give yourself credit for recognising it.* Even if criticism itself can be constructive, fear of criticism is likely to be unhelpful. To learn, we need to be able to accept advice in an open and uninhibited way. For this to be possible, we need to feel safe about making and noticing our mistakes. Children who are brought up in an environment where the response to making a mistake is ridicule or punishment are unlikely to allow themselves to think or act freely and creatively. A secure and supportive framework is essential for learning.

In dealing with fear, physical contact can be an important means of reassurance. Manual support and guidance is an effective teaching tool in swimming, but conventional teaching methods offer little constructive advice or training in such techniques. The usual environment for teaching swimming is one in which the teacher is an authority figure. Teachers and coaches conventionally carry out swimming instruction standing outside the water, shouting orders to groups of pupils with whom they have limited or no physical contact. From a child's perspective, the coach towers above, teaching by command rather than by example. The teacher's apparent aloofness can seem unsupportive and intimidating. Children may also be swept along by competitive peer pressures (as we described in Chapter 2, see p.51), thereby missing out on valuable lessons of confidence and safety; and group dynamics can mean that the individual child is forced to suppress his or her own fears and inadequacies so as not to be singled out. Much depends on the teacher's own skill and perceptiveness: there is no doubt that in many circumstances group teaching can be effective, as well as time-saving and cost-efficient. However, responsible one-to-one physical assistance in the water may be invaluable in giving a feeling of confidence and safety both to children and adult learners.[2]

All teachers agree that a sense of confidence in water is essential to swimming. However, insufficient attention is paid to the specific issues that must be addressed if the learner is to acquire

[2] Traditional methods of swimming-teaching do not provide instructors with the rationale or explicit techniques for giving pupils constructive physical support in the water. Concerns about abuse of children in particular has led to a climate in which swimming-teachers are discouraged from any kind of physical contact with young pupils. In teaching the *AT* (in or out of the water) the primary emphasis is

confidence. This neglect partly stems from thinking of swimming as a purely physical activity. It's assumed that the development of swimming skills alone is enough for the learner to become confident about the water. This is rarely the case. When skills are acquired without first establishing a sound basis of confidence, a crucial aspect of swimming is bypassed. This omission is at the expense of a whole dimension of sensitivity to being in the water and a more profound enjoyment of swimming. The situation may be illustrated by the following model:

Fig 3.5 *Traditional instructional model*

Lack of confidence ⟶ **Swimming skills** ◄·········► Confidence

It's true that acquiring competent motor skills leads to greater confidence in water, which in turn encourages the further development of such skills. The better you're able to move through water, the more confident you're bound to feel about being in the water. But your confidence will not be well grounded if it is treated merely as a by-product of skills, as the model illustrates. Supposing an unexpected situation arises – an attack of cramp or water splashing unexpectedly in your face. Well-practised motor skills can become inadequate or irrelevant. In the face of such an occurrence the first arrow swings round, and the pathway leads straight back to the initial situation – inability and fear. The fact that your swimming skills are based on inadequate foundations means there is a sense of precariousness and unease about the whole question of being in the water.

Far better, then, that teaching should include explicit instruction to establish confidence, both prior to and parallel with the development of motor skills in the water. This requires a shift of emphasis. The revised instructional model shows a teaching path which leads *via* confidence-building measures to the development of soundly based swimming skills:

Fig 3.6 *Revised instructional model*

Lack of confidence ⟶ **Confidence** ◄⟶ **Swimming skills**

on the head-neck-back relationship, and the use of the teacher's hands for guidance in this area means that swimming instruction with the *AT* is likely to be hands-on as well. The formulation of explicit guidelines on touch would be a helpful starting-point to make both teachers and pupils more aware of the appropriate boundaries.

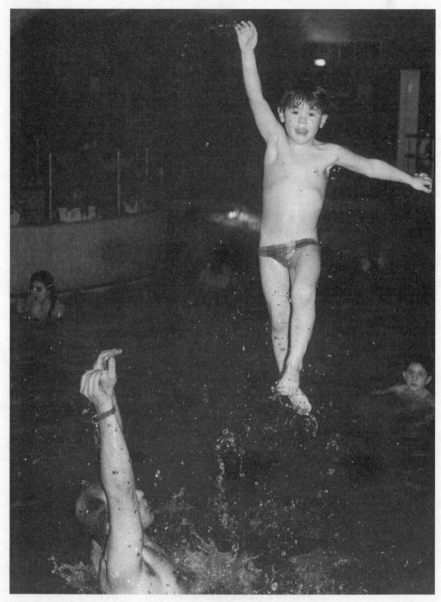

Fig 3.7
*Forward and up! Water confidence should be taught
alongside swimming skills.*

This model is a useful basis for thinking about the learning of
any skill. The educationist John Dewey saw the *AT* in a similar light,
as being an essential preliminary to the acquisition of learning. He

wrote that the *AT* "bears the same relation to education that education bears to all other human activities".

Tense Mind, Tense Body

What happens when we're afraid? Fear is far more than a purely psychological matter. In fact, it highlights the inseparability of the psychological and physiological domains. When we are afraid, anxious or worried, our whole body registers the response in a variety of ways. Expressions associated with fear include "seizing up" and "becoming rigid", a "sinking feeling" or a "knot in the stomach". Such reactions exemplify the characteristic sense of discomfort associated with feeling afraid. They have physiological correlates in the disposition of our musculo-skeletal structure and the release of chemicals into our bloodstream. These changes are not under our conscious control: the instruction "Don't be afraid" is surely asking a lot of someone who experiences fear in any normal sense!

All mammals have similar physiological reactions to the experience of danger or to its perceived threat. In this situation, a series of chemical impulses are triggered in the autonomic nervous system, resulting in instantaneous changes in the body. These include changes in the cardiovascular system, as adrenalin is produced to facilitate a burst of energetic movement; changes in the respiratory system – breathing becomes shallower and more rapid; and a temporary shutdown of the digestive system, to allow more energy to be transferred to the limbs. These reactions are the body's way of preparing to negotiate danger by fighting, freezing or running away. The exact nature of the changes and the way in which they are felt vary between species and individuals. Human beings associate the experience with sensations such as a pounding heart, sweating, dryness of the mouth, and a tightening of the chest. The effects can be clearly seen when people take fright: their bodies stiffen, their eyes widen, and the colour drains from the faces.

The difference between the fear response in human beings and in other mammals is that for animals the effects are short-lived and usually pass as soon as danger recedes. In humans they endure, and sometimes persist long after the threat has passed. In the case of a particularly traumatic event, psychophysical symptoms can persist for several days, weeks or even years. It's as if the experience remains trapped in our bodies. People who are scared of swimming often recall a particular episode in their past when they felt an acute sense of fear of being in water. The experience can have such a marked effect that the mere thought of swimming makes them extremely nervous. These fear responses are so ingrained that aquaphobes convince themselves that they will never be able to shake off their fear.

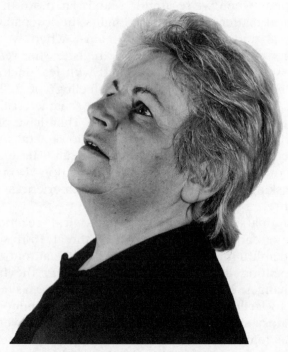

Fig 3.8
The startle reflex: the head jerks back and the eyes widen.

However, there is at least one aspect of our fear reactions which, once we are made fully aware of it, we can learn to bring under our conscious control to some degree. This is the *startle pattern*, the reflex at the core of the Alexander Technique, which was introduced in Chapter 1. When we receive a sudden shock – a loud noise or bright light in our faces, or an unexpected piece of bad news – we have a tendency to contract the muscles of our neck involuntarily, causing the head to be thrust backwards. Muscular reactions which accompany this reflex include raising our shoulders, tensing our arms, stiffening our chests, and flexing the leg muscles so that our knees lock. All this takes place within a split second. These reactions have evolved as an automatic defensive response in the face of danger, and therefore are extremely difficult, if not impossible, to avoid in most circumstances.

Although the most drastic manifestations of the startle pattern can be observed at moments of extreme tension, less pronounced forms can be detected in everyday situations. At home or at work, in public or in private, we are subjected to situations and events which can cause us to seize up with worry or apprehension. It can even happen when the phone rings! However, we can learn to exercise some conscious control so that the impact of the startle pattern is reduced and its effects do not linger. By cultivating a more balanced and aware disposition through the *AT*, we can prevent it taking place as often as it might, and to minimise its effects.

Some types of anxiety are so pronounced and incapacitating that they are considered serious psychological disorders, and are classified as phobias. These include fear of spiders (arachnophobia), of being enclosed (claustrophobia), or of public places (agoraphobia).[3] Specific treatments have been devised to help reduce or eliminate phobias. Cognitive therapies work on the premise that one first needs to examine and understand the irrational nature of one's fear in order to be released from it. Combined with behavioural techniques, such as gradual exposure to fear-inducing situations, they have proved particularly effective.

A different approach to the problem of 'mental blocks' was developed by Wilhelm Reich, a one-time student of Freud's. Reich believed that traumatic experiences remain fixed in our musculature. He identified the 'character-muscular armour' as the main obstacle to healthy psychological functioning. 'Character armour' consists of defensive character traits (such as debilitating shyness) developed in childhood as a way of warding off painful feelings. 'Muscular armour' is manifested in the muscular spasms which represent the bodily expression of these attitudes. Reich proposed a combination of psychotherapeutic and physical techniques to break down such emotional armouring and to release pent-up psychic and physical energies.

This approach has certain similarities to that adopted by the *AT*. However, the *AT* is less concerned with analysing the origins of fear than with learning to undo what Alexander called "overexcited fear

---

[3] Aquaphobia, commonly used to mean "fear of *swimming*", is rarely included in such classifications. Extreme dread of *water* is very rare: hydrophobia, where water is avoided even for drinking, is a symptom of rabies, and a life-threatening condition.

responses". In practice, remembering an early traumatic event related to swimming does little to help the inhibition of extreme psychophysical reactions that occur in or near a swimming-pool. Dwelling on negative experiences in the past can even increase the feeling of fear associated with swimming.

From the *AT* perspective, working directly with the fear *reactions* is the key to eradicating disabling symptoms of anxiety. This is achieved by first awakening a fuller awareness of the reactions themselves, and then showing how they can be mastered. Attention to the "means-whereby" – the best *use* of oneself in the present moment – is a remarkably effective way of removing an unproductive focus on the original source of anxiety. This involves a *redirection* of attention from the fear itself to the process involved in performing the activity (see, for example, Case Study 3 below). People who are afraid of water are rarely aware of their specific reactions to it. Armed with a new awareness of the obstacles they are creating for themselves, they can work effectively on letting go of the patterns of action into which they fall without thinking. In this way they can eventually discover for themselves that the water can be a safe, comfortable and enjoyable environment.

The practice of the Alexander Technique encourages a sense of continual exploration and self-discovery. Exploration requires the readiness to embrace the new in order to discover and experience the unknown. The *AT* challenges us to confront our fears by becoming aware of how habitual reactions limit us and prevent personal growth. The 'forward and up' of the *AT* is a movement that is both literal and symbolic: it represents leaving our fears behind and progressing to a higher level of thought and action in our daily lives.

Case Study 3: Amanda – Overcoming Aquaphobia

At 40, Amanda was a self-confessed aquaphobe. The thought of having to swim was enough to make her tremble and come out in a cold sweat. This she attributed to an early experience when she was thrown into deep water by a (so-called) swimming instructor. She recalled the event with great clarity, remembering in detail how she had felt at the time. She thought she was going to drown, and was pulled from the pool in a state of abject terror.

With great courage, Amanda decided to try to overcome her phobia by confronting her fear head-on. She enrolled on a course of group swimming lessons, but after several months had made very little progress. Although she was able to enter a shallow pool and propel herself for a short distance, the sense of panic persisted. Around the same time, she embarked on a series of *AT* lessons to help her deal with a chronic back condition. She was referred to an *AT* swimming instructor, who adopted a one-to-one approach that was radically different from her previous teacher's. Amanda's attention was drawn to her habitual response of tensing her neck and holding her breath. The teacher supported her head and neck as she lay on her back in the water, and gently pulled her along, ensuring that she was breathing easily and that her neck muscles remained free. After a few lessons she was able to float unaided, and proceeded to learn to perform the various strokes. Her most important lesson was that of *trust:* she had learned to trust first her teacher, then the water, and ultimately herself.

Facing the Water with Confidence

Whoever looks into the mirror of the water will see first of all his own face. Whoever goes to himself risks a confrontation with himself. The mirror does not flatter, it faithfully shows whatever looks into it...This confrontation is the first test of courage on the inner way, a test sufficient to frighten off most people.

Carl Jung

Not many people are afraid of putting their feet in water. Or their hands. Or their hips, their arms, their shoulders, their necks... But if there is a sticking-point, it is invariably the face. What is it about the face that makes it seem so vulnerable? In short, the eyes, nose, ears, and mouth! Despite all evidence to the contrary, many people behave as if simply submerging their face will subject its vital and sensitive orifices to intense discomfort or to the unstoppable influx of water. Is there any basis for such fears? Most swimmers would readily agree that such concerns are exaggerated. Nonetheless, whether or not rationally or even consciously held, they need to be thought about and addressed. They are obstacles to appreciating how the immersion of the face is a necessary, integral, and potentially greatly rewarding aspect of the art of swimming.

The eyes are undoubtedly delicate and sensitive organs. Most of us detest the sensation of medicinal drops being dripped into our eyes. When a foreign body touches the cornea, our automatic reaction is to blink and flicker our eyelids, and there's a natural tendency for the eye to water. These reflexes serve to protect the cornea from damage. With practice we can learn to 'inhibit' these reactions – an important ability if we wish to wear contact lenses, or to open our eyes under water unprotected by a mask or goggles. There are, of course, realistic concerns about the effect on our eyes of possible pollutants and detergent chemicals used to disinfect pools. But whilst prolonged exposure of the eyes to chlorine and other chemicals can cause irritation, in most swimming-pools the levels are carefully monitored and controlled so that the water is safe, even if swallowed by mistake.[4]

Anxiety that injury or pain to the eye might result from water alone being in contact with the cornea is misplaced. With its softness and neutral pH balance, water is a safe medium for the eyes. However, even when they keep their eyes tightly shut underwater, some swimmers feel the need to wipe water off their eyelids before they re-open them. The habit of using the hands to sweep the water constantly away from the eyes is often observed in beginners, but should be discouraged as it impedes learning to swim at any stage. Flicking the eyelashes and blinking the eyelids are all that is required for the eye to repel excess water. Familiarity with the feeling of water bathing the cornea – whether through regular swimming or practice in the bath (see box below) – helps to remove unnecessary and distracting concerns about getting water in the eyes.

Countering the fear of putting your face in water

1. Accept your fear. Don't try to deny it in any way or you will compound your difficulties.
2. Be patient with yourself. Don't put unnecessary pressure on yourself by trying to conquer the fear in a day. Recognise that it is deeply ingrained and may take time to undo.
3. Learn how to exhale confidently into the water (see Ch.5, p.136).
4. Pay attention to your orientation (see Ch.4, p.105). By redirecting your attention, you can gradually become more at ease with the way your face rests in the water.
5. Take every opportunity to wet your face – in the basin, bath or shower. Build your familiarity with the sensation of water in contact with all parts of your face – without resorting to rubbing it away from your eyes.

---

[4] People who are ultra-sensitive to chlorine or have allergic reactions to certain chemicals obviously need to take special care about chemically disinfected pools. Fortunately, there is a growing range of alternative methods of cleaning, filtering, and disinfecting pools.

Getting water in the ears is another distraction, but one which need not present excessive concern to swimmers. Reactions range from an irrational anxiety that simply placing the ears in the water will cause them to fill up, to an exaggerated worry about water remaining trapped inside the ears. The complex series of twists and turns inside the human ear effectively prevents water penetrating beyond its outer parts. The deeper, more delicate region towards the eardrum is virtually inaccessible. Occasionally water can be trapped by wax in the outer canals of the ear, causing temporary discomfort. If the water is allowed to remain there for an extended period, bacterial infection can develop, but inflammation is more often the consequence of excessive efforts to clear and dry the interior channels. Usually, water drains away of its own accord even if it has been trapped in the ear for a time.

In the case of both eyes and ears, it's not just the physical contact with water that can be the cause of anxiety. Often it's because their functions – seeing and hearing – seem to be affected or impaired. This is mainly because the aquatic environment presents different kinds of visual and aural stimuli to those we normally experience outside the water. Under the water, sounds are muffled and sights appear less distinct. Some sounds will seem magnified: one's own breathing and heartbeat, for instance. It's important not to be put off from exhaling strongly simply because it sounds louder than expected (see Chapter 5, p.136). These sensations should not provoke alarm: unfamiliarity alone makes them intimidating. With time and experience, we easily become accustomed to the different quality of sensations in and around the water, and adjust our expectations accordingly.

Fears of placing the nose and mouth in the water are largely related to fears about breathing, which are discussed in detail in Chapter 5. The question of how we breathe when swimming is of paramount importance to learning to feel at home in the water. The physiological mechanism known as the *oral seal* acts as an effective barrier to water getting into our lungs. We need to familiarise ourselves in practice with the operation of this mechanism, so that unnecessary fears do not overwhelm us and cause us to override it by our own undue efforts. Additionally there are a number of swimming accessories, discussed in the section below (p.86) which can be invaluable in helping swimmers overcome their fears about putting their face in the water.

Once we have learned to put our face in water, we stand to derive additional benefit from the effects of another remarkable physiological mechanism, known as the *dive instinct*. The dive instinct was first identified in seals, who despite being mammals are able to swim for extended periods under water. It was found that this ability is linked to a measurable change in their metabolism, which to a greater or lesser degree affects all mammals when the face is immersed in water. This change comprises a noticeable slow-down in the activity of the respiratory, digestive, and cardiovascular systems. The cumulative effect is to allow for a slower release of energy and accompanying feelings of tranquillity and release – that is, so long as negative thoughts do not interfere and counteract these effects. There are thus positive physiological and psychological benefits to be gained from conquering the fear of putting the face in the water. Those who choose to swim with their heads held clear of the water – often, in fact, because of unacknowledged fears – are missing out on the very experience that could help to put a different perspective on their feelings.

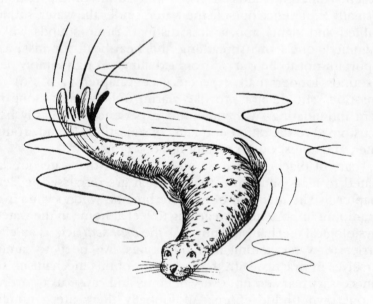

Fig 3.9
The seal: proud possessor of the dive instinct.

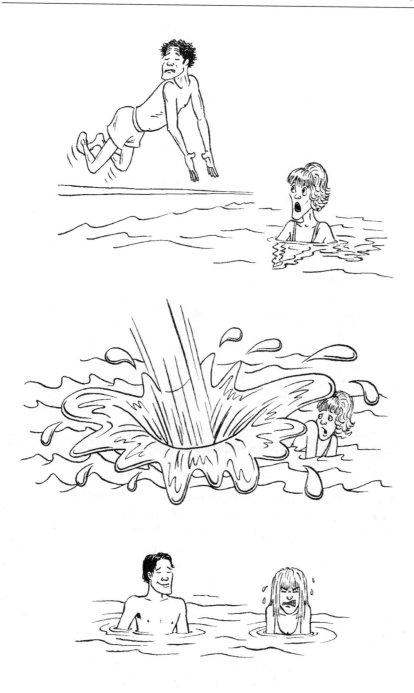

Fig 3.10
Swimming is not about keeping your hair dry!

Letting go of Fear

Apart from the specific fears mentioned above, people have more general anxieties about swimming. Some of the more common reasons – or excuses – people give for being put off swimming altogether are listed below. Can you identify with any of them? If you can, you may find that you also have reservations or unconscious mental blocks about dealing in a practical way with your difficulties. However, it helps to recognise exactly what needs to be addressed if it's going to present an obstacle to your feeling at home in the water. It can also help to be reassured that such thoughts are neither "silly" nor unique to you. You will find that in practice they are shared by many swimmers and non-swimmers. They have to be taken seriously, if only because – especially because – they are *your* feelings.

> ### *Thoughts that put us off swimming.*
>
> 1. The water will be uncomfortably cold/chlorinated.
> 2. The water will damage my hair/ruin my hairstyle.
> 3. I will be embarrassed showing my body in public.
> 4. The surroundings of the pool appear unhygienic.
> 5. My swimming style will be a source of ridicule.
> 6. I am unfit/my physique is unsuitable for swimming.
> 7. I will never be able to swim/swim well.

While some of these reflect an unwelcome reality which we may have to take practical measures to avoid or overcome, others such as nos. 6 and 7 are examples of mistaken beliefs – statements which may sound reasonable but in reality are not. For instance, virtually anyone can learn to swim – young, old, fat, thin, weak or strong. The belief that one will never be able to swim engenders a reluctance and rigidity which is counterproductive and can make the thought self-fulfilling. Such beliefs combine to create negative attitudes which constitute a major hindrance to progress. It's important that negative thoughts are not translated into destructive reactions. There are various techniques for countering negative thoughts. These include learning to "let go" of thoughts, repeating positive affirmations, and "creatively visualising" a desirable alternative. Whilst all these may be helpful, the *AT* approach can be distinguished from them. It simply proposes that you learn to be aware of, and inhibit, the automatic psychophysical reactions which accompany such beliefs. The resulting self-awareness encourages you to explore and discover *any* form of solution which you personally find creative and beneficial.

You can usefully experiment with practical ways which appeal to you of overcoming negative thoughts and diminishing the discomfort involved with the very idea of swimming. We have made a number of suggestions in this chapter, based on ideas of becoming *familiar* with new and initially uncomfortable sensations, *exploring* practical solutions to overcoming anxiety, becoming *aware* of habitual reactions, and *redirecting* attention to use rather than dwelling on negative thoughts. These techniques conveniently enough form an acronym:

Familiarity **E**xploration **A**wareness **R**edirection

By bearing these ideas in mind, you can turn unproductive anxieties into practical steps to overcoming them. What were *reasons* for avoiding swimming become *excuses*. The challenges vary enormously between different individuals. Accept the challenge and create your own solutions.

Exploring the Water

Learning has to be an adventure, otherwise it's stillborn. What you learn at a given moment ought to depend on chance meetings, and it ought to continue in that way, from encounter to encounter, a learning in transformations, a learning in fun.

Elias Canetti

Just as play is an important part of how children learn, exploration and a sense of fun are an important part of adult learning. Swimming doesn't have to be serious and solemn, or conform to rigid rules and procedures. Below we suggest some ways of exploring the water, once you are familiar with putting your face in it. They should be performed with appropriate supervision (depending on your level of ability) and in an environment which allows you the freedom to do it (not, for example, a crowded racing pool!). Think of them as starting-points for your own exploration.

Experiment, adapt, innovate, and find your own ways of being free in the water.

Floating
Find out what the water can do for you, and what it actually feels like. On your front, on your back, on your side, and alternating, discover how your own body works in relation to the water. See what happens when you make yourself deliberately tense or relaxed, with your head and limbs in different positions, lying motionless, or gliding after pushing off from the side.

Underwater
Experience what it's like to sink feet-first, or to plunge head-first underwater, to rest on the bottom of the pool holding your breath and breathing out slowly, and to swim along under the water. Try propelling yourself underwater in different ways, e.g. using just the legs, performing a dolphin kick (legs straight, bending at the knees and kicking back together). Note how much effort is required not to rise to the surface! Savour the meditative solitude of being totally surrounded by water.

Twists and Twirls
As you manoeuvre in the water without a set direction or goal, you can learn a lot about balance and how the weight of your head affects your movements. Become familiar with the working of the oral seal: see how easily you are able to inhale when your face is above the surface, and to avoid inhaling when it is under water.

Technical aids and accessories

Because a sense of ease in the water is so essential to the art of swimming, equipment that helps to promote this is a worthwhile investment. Adults who have difficulty putting their face in the water for any length of time can find good-quality swimming accessories invaluable. As the majority of swimming-pools use chlorine as a disinfectant (and even lakes and oceans may contain eye irritants), the eyes are likely to sting if they stay open underwater for long periods. To help prevent this, there's no substitute for a pair of good, well-fitting goggles. Without them, many swimmers will prefer to close their eyes the majority of the time. This not only increases the risk of bumping into things such as walls, lane ropes and other swimmers, but more importantly it contributes to a feeling of nervousness and of being in an alien environment. This is particularly true for swimmers who have poor eyesight to begin with. Straining one's eyes to see the end of a pool or to avoid obstacles is not conducive to feeling at home in the water!

For some swimmers, goggles feel uncomfortably tight or constricting and seem to leak and fog up constantly. In the box below, we make suggestions for ways of overcoming such concerns. Today there are hundreds of different makes of goggles on the market, and it's worth getting a pair that offers maximum effectiveness with minimum discomfort. There should be no gaps between the eyepieces and the flesh around your eyes. Our faces are all different shapes and sizes: if you have a small face, for instance, choose goggles which taper inward and hug its contours tightly. Goggles should be easily adjustable across the nose, and preferably have a double strap to hold them firmly in place, so that the pressure around the back of the head is even. If necessary, they can be ordered with lenses made to your prescription.

Some points about goggles

1. When fitting goggles, first place the strap at the back of your head. Bring the eyepieces in front of your eyes and adjust the goggles so that they fit firmly over your face.
2. If the goggles leak from the inside corners, adjust the width of the nose-strap; if from the outside, tighten the strap around your head. It helps to create a slight vacuum in front of the eyes to ensure that the goggles are watertight. You should expect the goggles to feel very tight when you are outside the water. They will feel less tight when you are swimming, because they will be partially buoyed up by water.
3. Goggles that are pre-treated with an anti-fog coating should not be taken off and rinsed at frequent intervals, as this doesn't give the chemicals a chance to work to disperse the fogging.
4. Expect to take time in fitting goggles correctly and getting used to them. It's worth persevering as they can substantially improve the quality of your experience of swimming.

Apart from goggles, a number of accessories are widely available to help swimmers deal with their concerns. It's worth considering anything that serves to prevent distraction, difficulty, or genuine discomfort. A swimming cap is a boon for swimmers with long hair, and may be essential to prevent waterlogged hair flopping over the eyes and mouth. Although you may have to accept that they are uncomfortable and not always totally effective in keeping the hair dry, their main purpose is to keep hair out of your face so that you can attend to your swimming. Water-tight ear-plugs are helpful for swimmers prone to ear infections or who suffer earache when the head is underwater. However, they can add to a sense of isolation in the water. Similarly, nose-clips are not recommended unless you have specific sinus problems, because they're likely to prevent you learning the appropriate ways of breathing when you swim. For hair and skin, shampoos and gels are widely available to neutralise chemicals and remove the smell of chlorine.

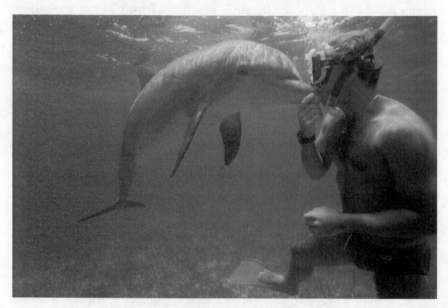

Fig 3.11
*Human beings are privileged to be able to
relate to friendly, intelligent dolphins.*

Conclusion

Asked what the single most important factor is in learning to swim, most people would reply "Confidence". A sense of trust – what we have called being at home in the water – provides the foundation for us to do whatever else might come naturally in the water. As we have seen, floating, propelling ourselves, and avoiding the intake of water into our lungs are all things which *do* come naturally to us in the earliest period of our lives. It's a shame that so many people are prevented from capitalising on these natural abilities, and learn instead to be fearful or anxious about water. However, with the right approach and support, confidence and ease in the water can be learned afresh.

We have suggested that elements of fear are present in most swimmers to a greater or lesser degree. Its effects range from an obvious and debilitating awkwardness to a reluctance to engage in a wholehearted exploration of the water's potential for pleasure. It's true that human beings are not like fishes or dolphins: water is not the medium in which we live. But it is more natural to us than we often allow. If water can never actually be our home, in developing the art of swimming we are discovering ways in which we can become more at home in the water than we might ever have imagined we could.

4. *Leading with the Head: Orientation & Balance*

Gravity is the root of lightness; stillness is the ruler of movement.

Lao Tzu

In nature, things tend upward. More precisely, living organisms have an observable tendency to grow and strive *forward, upward and outward*. Life is a continuous dynamic process, and this is one of the complex ways in which living things, including human beings, respond to nature's laws. The force of gravity is a feature of the world which both keeps us with our feet on the ground and gives us the wherewithal to grow upwards. Although gravity seems to bear down on us relentlessly, life on earth also flourishes *because* of gravity. It allows us to develop healthily, helping to shape and form our bodies like wood turned on a lathe. In a weightless environment plants grow misshapen and poorly: it's as if they have lost their natural sense of direction.

This upward sense of direction, or **orientation**, separates the living from the dead, the organic from the inert, the healthy from the sick. It exists on many levels: conscious and unconscious, physical and psychological, literal and metaphorical. The inclination towards positive growth is a defining element of human nature, balanced by a desire to maintain our equilibrium through change. But every moment of our lives we are subject to, and often actively resist, forces which threaten to unbalance us and pull us down. All change involves a degree of destabilisation. The *AT* offers practical guidance in handling these competing forces within and without. At the core of the Technique is the insight that how we orient ourselves – the basis of good *use* – is intimately connected with our mental and physical responses to the environment. The practice of the *AT* helps us to discover a better orientation and balance, with far-reaching consequences both for the way we move and for how we choose to lead our lives.

How are orientation and balance connected? They are really the same thing, looked at from a different perspective. Visualise a pair of scales. At rest it consists of two basic elements in dynamic

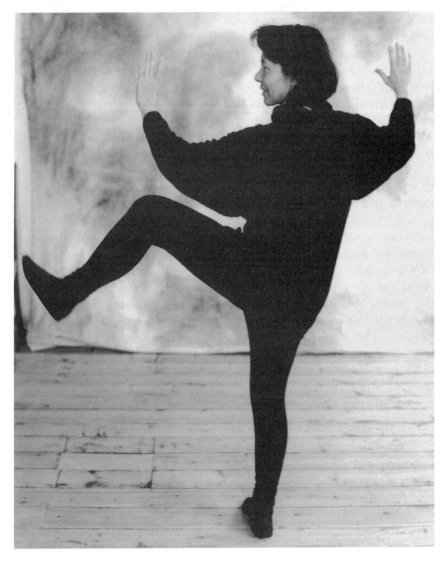

Fig 4.1
In Tai Chi, orientation and balance unite.

opposition to each other – the fulcrum and the beam. They can only function properly when the base provides a steady central balancing-point. The beam rests in equilibrium on a fulcrum that exerts a countervailing upward force. A change in the position of the base requires a corresponding adjustment of the beam. This image can be applied to the way our bodies work as we move: the spine provides the upward thrust that allows our upper body to balance naturally, in continuous fluid realignment as we move. Orientation and balance are two sides of the same coin.

Although primarily conceived as aspects of our physique, the ideas of orientation and balance have broader implications. If we live with constant physical imbalance, the chances are that we will grow mentally unbalanced as well. A sense of orientation grounds us as living organisms and allows for balanced growth and change. Thus the healthy response to our physical environment lays the basis for a healthy outlook on life.

The ideas of orientation and balance have great significance for the art of swimming. Water offers us a special medium in which to explore the way we use ourselves. Because swimming is performed in a horizontal plane, gravity acts on our body in a different way from when we walk upright. It is also counteracted by the water's buoyancy. This can act as an aid, if we allow it, to giving us a sense of a beneficial forward-and-outward orientation. Conversely, if we resist the natural properties of the water in relation to our bodies, the problems resulting from our poor use are magnified; we will find it hard to move or to swim with any degree of real pleasure or success. The habit of pulling the head back and down may pass completely unnoticed in our daily activities. However, the same tendency when swimming has immediate and substantial effects which are hard to ignore. The environment of water offers a greater opportunity to observe the effects of changes in our orientation.

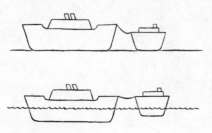

Fig 4.2
On land, the cable (neck) which joins the tugboat (head) to the liner (torso) is at a different angle to when both are buoyed up by the water.

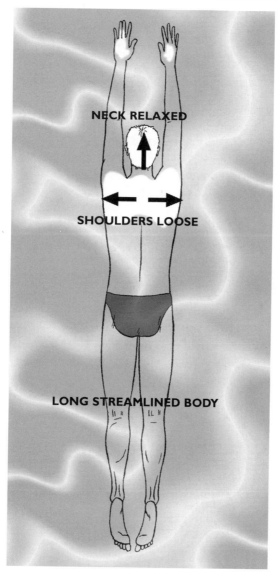

Fig 4.3(a)
A well-oriented body in any plane is directed forwards and outwards...

The exact way in which we orientate ourselves to best effect differs between individuals. A 'right' position does not exist. It should also be reiterated that the forces and pressures acting on the body in the water differ in important respects from those which operate outside it. In particular, the buoyancy of water means that

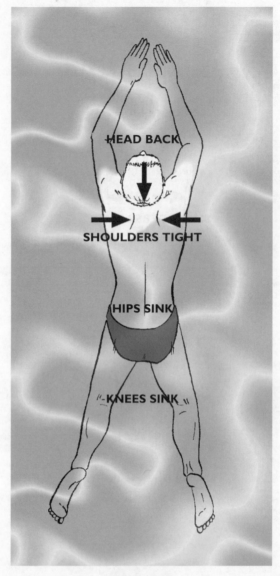

HEAD BACK

SHOULDERS TIGHT

HIPS SINK

KNEES SINK

Fig 4.3(b)
rather than backwards and inwards.

the natural alignment of the head, neck and back is likely to be subtly different from good orientation when we walk or stand upright. Outside the water, releasing the neck encourages an upright axis of the head. But what happens if we release our neck when we rest prone on the water? Buoyancy affects the angle of the head, so that even when we release our neck the head is inclined *slightly further back* than when we walk upright on dry land. Underwater, the balance of surrounding forces encourages a different, straighter orientation yet again (look at the swimmers depicted on the Front Cover). But if we wanted to adopt, when swimming the crawl for instance, the same 'posture' as we present when standing erect, we might have to apply unnecessary effort to keep our head tucked in. The aesthetic criteria whereby good orientation is assessed must take this factor into account.

Notice, for example, how the good orientation of the champion *runner* differs from that of the champion *swimmer* (see Fig 4.4).

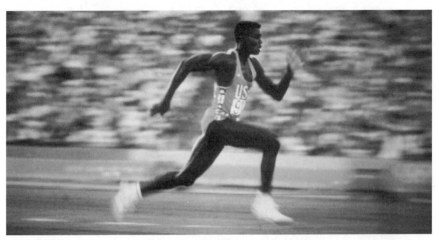

Fig 4.4
*Carl Lewis and Andy Jameson: champion runner and swimmer show
how different activities require different orientations.*

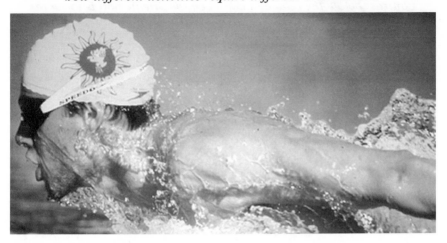

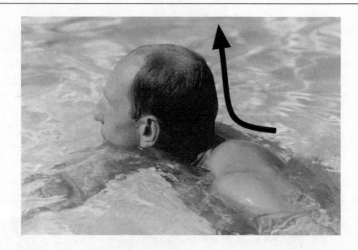

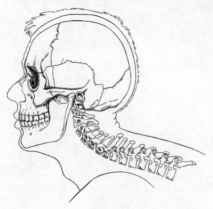

Fig 4.5
Swimming with the head back, the vertebrae are compressed.
Contrast below the relaxed neck when the orientation is forward.

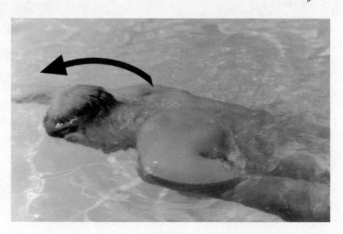

The tendency to let the head tilt back, encouraged by buoyancy, should not be confused with fixing the muscles of the neck so that the head is unduly jammed back. In practice, you have to discover for yourself the balance that allows you to swim with freedom and efficiency. A practical understanding of orientation and balance in the water enables us to explore our own relationship to the water, and brings us closer to attaining ease and efficiency when swimming. The new awareness gained from our experience in water can also be extended to our experience outside the water. In this way we can gain a vital insight into the importance of orientation and balance in our daily lives.

Explore how changes in your orientation affect you in the water. Push off from the wall face down, with your neck free and your head leading your body in a forward-and-up orientation. Now sharply contract the muscles of your neck so that your head is pulled up out of the water. Observe how this causes the lower back to arch, so that your hips and legs sink and start to drag you down.

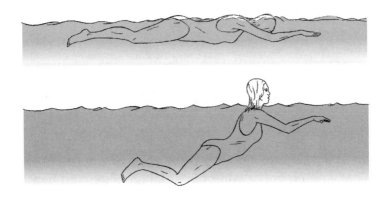

Fig 4.6
Raising the head encourages the lower body to sink immediately.

Orientation and the AT

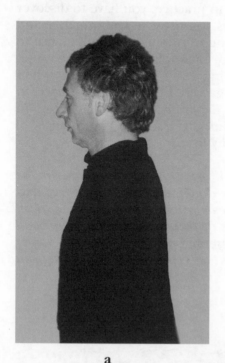
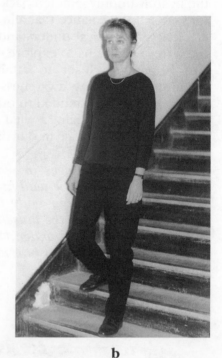

a   b

Fig 4.7
a) Relaxing upwards. b) Walking down but thinking up.

The dynamic relationship between the head, neck and back plays a
crucial role in the way we orient ourselves. The main element of use
that determines our ease of movement is the poise of our head in
relation to the rest of the body. With the head as the leading
element of a forward-and-upward orientation, there is a freeing of
the spinal column and a consequent lengthening and widening of
the torso which facilitates good breathing and generally balanced
movement. In the *AT* the head-neck-back relationship is seen as
central in promoting good use and healthy functioning (which is
why F.M. Alexander termed it *the primary control*.) The operation
of the primary control can be clearly observed in the easy poise
shown by infants and animals.

As we grow older, the delicate balance which characterises the
natural relationship between head, neck and back deteriorates. We
acquire the habit of contracting our neck muscles as a defensive

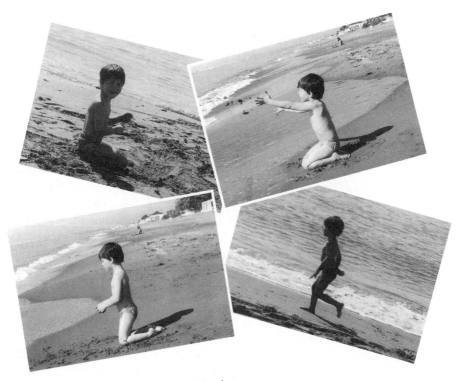

Fig 4.8
Children show natural balance and poise.

response to unpleasant stimuli. This stiffening of the neck causes
the head to be forced back and down, which works against the natural extension of our spinal column. Our vertebrae are compressed,
like a line of railway carriages being shunted together when the
brakes are applied at the front. This is the first in a chain of reactions which combine to create tension throughout the body and
interfere with our ease of movement. Ultimately the spine is connected by nerves and muscles to every part of the body. When the
spine loses its upward orientation and contracts, the back loses its
function as our basic support structure. This creates undue strain
on other parts of the body, and we seek to compensate for it by
"holding ourselves up". Our whole musculo-skeletal structure is
affected. Our ribcage becomes compressed, constricting the breathing mechanism. Our shoulders are narrowed, hampering the freedom of the arms. The pelvic region is put under pressure, affecting
the ability of the legs to move with ease. The first step to reversing
all these effects is to stop the unnecessary contraction of the

Fig 4.9

With the head pulled back, muscular tension extends throughout the body. This cross-section dramatically illustrates how a position held by swimmers for extended periods would be impossible outside the water.

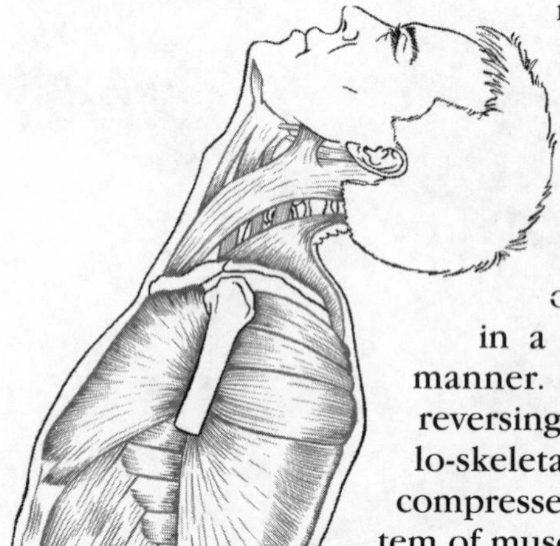

muscles of the neck so that our head-neck-back relationship can begin to improve. By freeing the point at which the head is connected to the rest of the body, the muscles of the torso are organised so that they interact in a more efficient and balanced manner. Tension is redistributed, reversing the contraction of the musculo-skeletal system that narrows and compresses the body. Because the system of muscles and bones involved is not normally under our direct conscious control, establishing the primary control is less about *doing* something to change than *allowing* internal musculo-skeletal structures to release. This is not a purely physical process: it also involves changing the way we think about ourselves. This connection is clear when we consider how emotions such as fear are regularly reflected in posture. A habitual attitude of worry or anxiety causes people to adopt a hunched, defensive stoop, while a positive, confident attitude has corresponding effects on use. We all know from experience how physical strain or discomfort affects our general outlook. Equally, emotions such as anxiety or anger produce muscular responses which increase tension throughout the body.

The *AT* respects the fact that mind and body form a psychophysical whole: change in one is reflected by change in the other. True flexibility in our physical aspect helps us to be more flexible on every level. This is not to be mistaken for the limited kind of flexibility which arises from training muscles to ignore pain when the body is distorted into extreme positions, whether in Yoga or in stretch-and-tone routines. Learning to change one's use is itself a dynamic process. It's not merely a question of re-adjusting one's *posture*, so that one holds oneself in a different position. For this reason F.M. Alexander cautioned against using the word 'posture', and words like 'position' and 'stance' are avoided in the *AT.* The quest for a better posture can all too easily lead to increased rigidity: the adoption of a fixed stance cannot be achieved without muscular tension. The classic 'upright' posture of the sergeant-major – head and shoulders back, chest out, tummy pulled in – was justly described by Alexander as "an abomination!" (see Fig 1.7, p. 31). It cannot be sustained without causing lasting injury to the spine. Constantly varying demands are made on our minds and bodies by the changing environments in which we find ourselves. In this context, no fixed posture can be appropriate: what's required is an *orientation* that allows for a truly flexible response.

Establishing the primary control is not a one-off action. Good orientation involves a living awareness of use that is renewed from moment to moment. Unless we're aware of our use, the inevitable tendency is to slip back into familiar patterns of thought and action. For instance, most of us make far too much effort in our daily lives. Look at the range of our basic daily activities: standing up and sitting down, walking, bending, dressing ourselves, brushing our teeth, lifting small objects. These can be performed with the minimum of muscular effort; but how often we find that they're done with an unnecessary level of accompanying strain and muscular tension! In focussing on a desired result, we all too often ignore the actual *process* which brings it about. The single-minded pursuit of goals elicits an automatic response to over-exert ourselves. We rarely stop to ask how much effort is really needed, or how it might best be directed.

Because the intermediate steps to our goal – the process of action – is where effort is unnecessarily expended, one way of ensuring that we save our energy and only exert ourselves appropriately is to be constantly aware of our use during the action. The only way we can do this effectively is to be aware of our use even before we act. In this way, good orientation is the essential preparation for the efficient performance of any action. The specific method proposed by the *AT* to help us prepare ourselves so that we avoid slipping into unhelpful habits is to repeat instructions to ourselves which guide us towards better use. F.M. Alexander devised a series of messages or 'orders' to be given in a continuous sequence, both as a prelude to and in the course of performing an action. The sequence of orders runs: "*Let the neck be free, to let the head go forward and up, to let the back lengthen and widen*". This is not an instruction for performing a finite course of tasks, but acts as a running prompt for achieving all the elements of good orientation simultaneously.[1] It is phrased in a way ("let" rather than "make") which emphasises that this is not about trying to perform specific actions. Rather, it's a way of stimulating us to *stop interfering* with the processes which allow us to be free. The projection of these messages "one after the other and all together" (in Alexander's words) makes us conscious of our use, and offers us a *means whereby* we can direct attention to improving our orientation.

Thus good orientation conveys the idea of a continually flexible forward-and-upward alignment of the head, neck and back, as a foundation for all further action. Patrick MacDonald, a graduate of Alexander's first teacher training course, has illustrated the concept of orientation in a vivid way: "*Even though a piece of steel does not move in space towards the magnet, every particle of the steel will be oriented towards it. While keeping the orientation of the particles towards the magnet it is possible to move both the magnet and the steel in any direction, including the opposite direction to which the particles are orientated.*" An example of this is how we can direct our body forward and up while at the same time, by bending at the hips and knees, bring it nearer to the ground (continuing to *think* forward and up).

Orientation in the Water

Thinking in activity requires attention and practice, but its application has a radical effect on the way we move and function. It is the key to breaking old habits and establishing a new way of acting. It also offers the means of developing the freedom and balance essential to the art of swimming. Balance here refers not simply to the physical aspect of our relationship to the water. It includes the idea of balanced integration of all the diverse elements of the activity. A balanced approach will prevent us, for instance, placing undue emphasis on any specific goal we have in mind to the

---

[1] At one time Alexander's word for these mental instructions was "directions". He also used "direction" to refer to *orientation*. We have avoided talking about 'direction' and 'directions' in contexts where confusion might arise between these distinct meanings.

detriment of our overall ability to swim.

One way in which good orientation helps very directly is by bringing about a reduced resistance of the water against the body – in other words, making the body more *streamlined*. Conventional swimming instruction, especially in competitive coaching, lays great emphasis on the streamlining of the body. It is rightly considered to be one of the most important factors in stroke efficiency. It's clear why this is: you can make tremendous efforts with your arms and legs to combat the water's resistance, but if you're poorly streamlined you will find it hard to move through the water. The position of your body will act as a brake to forward propulsion.

Case Study 4A: John – Using the Head in Swimming

John was a fitness enthusiast who regularly swam the breast stroke with his head out of the water. Despite exerting great force his progress through the water was frustratingly slow. The main reason was that the position of his head acted as a barrier to forward movement, so the power of his leg-kick was impeded. The majority of swimmers who keep their heads aloft do so out of fear. John had no such anxiety; he simply did not appreciate that releasing his neck and using the weight of his head to help him extend forward would significantly improve his streamlining and his ability to move.

He discovered that simply *letting go* of his neck muscles enabled him to achieve tremendous forward momentum without applying any more effort than usual. Because he was not afraid to experiment and adapt his style, in a short time had halved the number of strokes that it took him to swim the length of the pool.

However, swimmers can take the pursuit of a streamlined body to undesirable extremes. For example, competitive breast-strokers are often advised to round their shoulders so that their body offers the least possible surface area as it pushes forward through the water. While this may give an advantage of speed at competitive level, it does so at the cost of healthy use both in and out of the water. The cumulative effect of regularly narrowing and stretching the torso is for the shoulders to droop and the chest to collapse. Such effects persist well beyond the swimming session itself. Once we start to discover a more sensitive awareness of the use of our selves, it's clear that the attainment of extreme speed cannot be the only or indeed the main goal of swimming. The desire for excessive speed is itself a symptom of the unbalanced approach to goals of no intrinsic value that characterises much of modern life. The pursuit

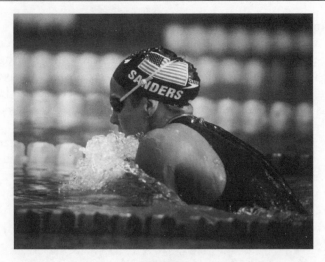

Fig 4.10
Hunching the shoulders in competitive breast stroke.

of speed *per se* is a prime example of how end-gaining can have undesirable side-effects on use.

Efficient swimming is a matter of using the optimum amount of energy to propel ourselves through the water. This requires two elements: reducing the water's resistance (or "drag") against our body, and applying propulsive force in the most economic manner. Good orientation – rather than forcing our body into a more streamlined shape – is the key to achieving a constructive balance of these elements. The elimination of unnecessary muscular tension in the body encourages us to float more easily.[2] When the body floats higher and flatter in the water, it offers less surface area for resistance. By promoting freedom in the joints and muscles, good orientation allows our limbs to engage with the water with greater control. It increases our sensitivity to where and when force should be applied most appropriately for the purpose of propulsion.

Note that forward-and-up orientation along the spine can take place on any plane – vertical, horizontal, or diagonal. The idea of orientation is not restricted to the upright plane. Furthermore, upward extension by itself is only one element of orientation. An equally important aspect is the process of *broadening* that naturally

---

[2] There is a surprisingly prevalent misconception that without sufficient forward momentum the body is bound to sink. Whilst speed can assist buoyancy, it can do so at the cost of good orientation.

accompanies the lengthening unless we prevent it in any way. For this reason, the attempt to stretch ourselves forcefully when swimming is misguided. Unduly narrowing the body interferes with the freedom and ease promoted by release and opening-out. When we swim, we can use the buoyancy of water to discover a whole range of different angles and positions in which our bodies can operate with ease. Water enables us to increase the spectrum of opportunities to experience good orientation within an environment that encourages us to move continuously. Holding our bodies stiffly limits our openness to such an experience. The art of swimming requires a constant, flexible adaptation of our bodies to conditions of buoyancy and liquidity.

Using Your Head

Freeing the neck and back allows the ribcage and diaphragm to work comfortably, permitting us to breathe in an unrestricted way. This promotes greater natural buoyancy and allows us to control the rhythm of our inhalation and exhalation (the rhythm of breathing, which is vital for good swimming, will be explored in the next chapter). A properly balanced body reduces the amount of effort required to prevent our legs and hips from dragging us down.

You can explore how buoyancy encourages a sense of good orientation by standing in calm water with your body submerged up to your chin. The pressure of the water supports the spine and allows you to stand without straining, your head free to pivot on the topmost vertebra.

The principle of good orientation shows once again that swimming requires us to be confident about putting our face in the water. Without this confidence, we're likely to interfere with our natural head-neck-back relationship. Is it possible to maintain good orientation if we swim with our head held clear of the water? Perhaps it is, but only for short periods: those who swim with their heads out of the water for long periods are not only subjecting their spines to damaging pressure, they're also hampering the process of lengthening and widening. And people who regularly swim in this way invariably complain of stiff necks and aching backs.

However, it's not enough just to put your face in the water: in itself this does not constitute good orientation. Even when the face is submerged below the water the head can remain jammed back against the shoulder girdle. But good orientation cannot occur *without* the neck muscles remaining free. This means that in the prone strokes (i.e. when we swim on our front) the head must be allowed to tilt forward under its own weight, leading to the lengthening and widening of the back and torso.[3]

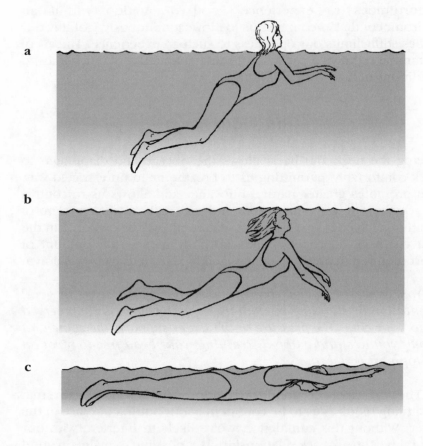

Fig 4.11
(a)With the head pulled back, the strain is obvious.
Even with the face submerged (b), swimming can be a strain
unless the orientation is forward (c).

[3] It may be necessary in a crowded pool to look ahead from time to time, but this can be done in such a way that elements of good orientation are preserved.

You can discover for yourself the importance of the head's counterpoise by exploring the effects of raising it in the water. Try the following set of manoeuvres for recovering your footing in the shallow end of a pool. Raising the head is the first stage of recovery, because it dramatically changes the body's orientation. This procedure is particularly important for beginners and those who lack confidence in recovering an upright position in shallow water after a glide.

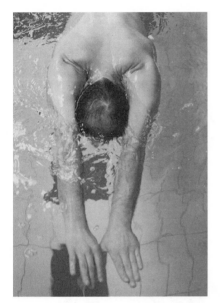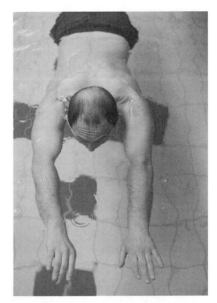

Fig 4.12
View from above: note the furrowed brow of the swimmer craning his head back to look ahead.

Breathing presents a challenge for maintaining good orientation in the water. If we were able, like seals or dolphins, to submerge ourselves for extended periods without breathing, it might be easier to maintain a balanced head-neck-back relationship. But we need to inhale through our nose or mouth more regularly. And because this means our face must surface above the water, learning to incorporate it into our stroke without interfering with good orientation is an important aspect of the art of swimming. Attempts are often made to side-step this problem. Medical professionals, even while recommending swimming for health, often advise against prone strokes – breast stroke or front crawl – for this reason.

1. *Push off from the side of the pool, hands out in front, with your head in the water leading your body forward.*
2. *Lift your head up and notice what happens to your body. It's as if you have applied the brake. Notice how your hips start sinking immediately.*
3. *Push forward with your arms to bring your torso towards the vertical.*
4. *Thrust your feet towards the ground.*

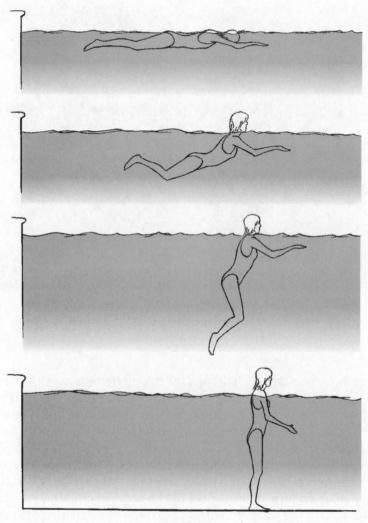

Fig 4.13

But the back stroke has its own complexities for maintaining good orientation. Some people think snorkels are the answer, but that merely limits the possibilities of the swimmer's art. In fact, it's far more rewarding to meet the challenge creatively, and thereby to expand rather than curtail your experience of swimming. There's great pleasure in discovering that it's possible to swim all the strokes *and* breathe well – without the use of props.

Aspects of Balance

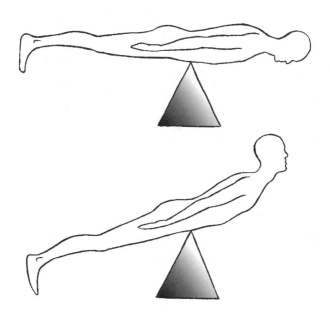

Fig 4.14
The human see-saw: how our head affects our longitudinal balance.

Good orientation in the water requires a continuous, flowing sense of balance. As we use our limbs to propel us through the water, the point of balance changes constantly. Holding the head in a fixed position interferes with this dynamic process. The point of balance at any one time depends on the relative positions of the various parts of the body, which are constantly changing as we move. One of the keys to discovering the art of swimming is a keen awareness of the delicate balance of our bodies in the water. Such an awareness provides the basis for ease and grace of movement, the distinguishing mark of the accomplished swimmer.

The body has a natural symmetry. Its weight is more or less equally distributed on either side of the spine. When we swim, the use of our limbs can either impede or assist the maintenance of our natural balance. If we pull harder with one arm without noticing it, we not only affect our ability to swim in a straight line, but disturb our overall poise. Similarly, uneven or uncoordinated use of the legs, which can be observed in swimmers who exhibit a "screw-kick" in the breast stroke, reduces our control of how we move through the water.

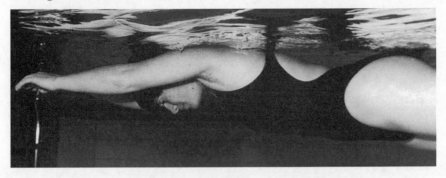

Fig 4.15
Just below the water surface , the head and arms forming a perfect counterpoise to the body as it glides forward.

In addition to these aspects of *lateral* balance, our body needs to find a dynamic equilibrium along its *length*. As with a see-saw, the weight of the head acts as an effective counterpoise to the downward pressure of the pelvic area. If we let go of our neck muscles when we lie prone on the water, our head naturally tends forward under its own weight. Rather than resist this tendency, we should learn to allow it to work in our favour when we swim.

Case Study 4B: Linda – Shifting the Balance

Linda, an accomplished swimmer, particularly enjoyed the front crawl for the sensation of speed and power. However, her experience was that she needed to kick with tremendous vigour. This alone seemed to prevent her legs sinking and dragging her body down. As a result, she was worn out after short periods of the crawl, and would relax by swimming other less energetic strokes.

In applying the *AT*, she learned to free her neck and back and lean forward into the water. As a result her balance shifted: legs and hips floated more easily, reducing the need for her to kick so hard to keep them up. She also became aware of another helpful effect: the widening of her torso helped her to breathe more fully, which improved her buoyancy and enabled her to release the muscles of her problematic lower back. These factors combined to transform her swimming style. In addition to speed and power, she gained a sense of rhythm and flow. She found that she could swim the crawl faster and for much longer periods without the usual feelings of strain and fatigue.

Conclusion

Most approaches to swimming emphasise the importance of body position and streamlining. As this chapter has shown, the concept of *orientation* is broader and its implications for the art of swimming are more far-reaching. In its widest aspect, orientation is about the way we think, act, and live, both in the water and outside it.

If we stop to think about our reasons for swimming, subjecting the body to the potentially damaging strains which result from poor orientation is unlikely to be one of them. But nowadays, as we discussed in Chapter 2, swimming is dominated by competitive goals. Technical procedures treat parts of the body in isolation, instead of starting with an awareness of how our organism works as a whole. Instruction is based on measures for achieving speed: performance in the water is judged by one's ability to get from *A* to *B* in the fastest possible time. Enjoyment, health and well-being are rarely the primary considerations. Principles of swimming developed for the competitive environment filter down to swimming-teaching at all levels. Efficiency is judged in purely external, quantitative terms, rather than our quality of experience.

But what is done in the pursuit of extreme speed is not always healthy or appropriate. Speed is just one aspect of swimming: focussing on it exclusively shows a lack of balance. It's hard to find a single photograph of an Olympic sprint-swimmer in action which doesn't show the neck muscles unduly tensed and the head fixed back. Yet it's clear that such a position militates against the most effective use of the self. For the recreational swimmer, an unbalanced approach based on the end-gaining attitude of the

Olympic competitor denies a whole range of possibilities that swimming has to offer. In particular, it obscures our potential for developing a healthier orientation – not only to swimming, but to life as a whole. The principles of the *AT* open our eyes to a radically different approach to swimming, one which integrates efficiency and elegance with balance and health. This approach fosters a new aesthetic for swimming style, and offers us the opportunity to re-appraise what constitutes the *art* of swimming.

STROKE GUIDE I:
Exploring orientation.

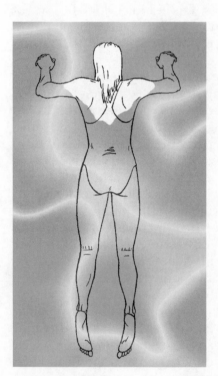 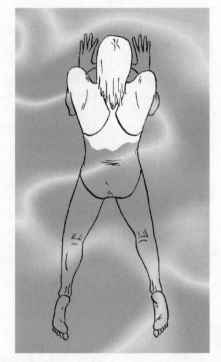

Fig 4.16 Phase 1
a) Arms – pull back.
b) Legs open and bend at the knee: raise head to inhale.

Different strokes require different skills. But while each stroke has its own particular features, all the strokes equally require that attention is paid to the principles of orientation. The ways in which we use our body in performing the various strokes raise distinctive challenges for the maintenance of good orientation. An attitude of exploration keeps the process alive: the purpose of technical practices is not to make you more rule-bound, but more free.

Breast Stroke

Efficient breast stroke can be divided, broadly speaking, into two phases: Movement and Rest. These elements of doing and non-doing need to be finely balanced for the stroke to be performed with fluidity and rhythm.

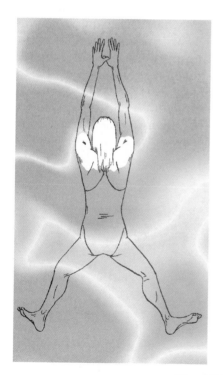 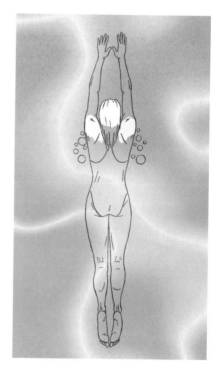

Fig 4.16 Phase 2
c) Kick back and draw legs together: head forward
d) Release: exhale: lengthen and widen

For purposes of illustration, this scheme somewhat oversimplifies the application of *AT* principles. In particular, it should be clear that the extension and release associated with good orientation need to be taking place *all the time*, in Phase 1 as well as Phase 2. Nonetheless, in breast stroke in particular, the ebb and flow of action and non-action is apparent. A common obstacle to swimming the breast stroke efficiently stems from a misunderstanding of the function of the arms. This is the only stroke in which the arms remain below the water-surface throughout, which limits the swimmer's ability to exert *propulsive* force with the arms. You therefore need to appreciate that the main propulsive force in the stroke is generated by leg action. Over-emphasising the role of the arms sometimes causes swimmers to perform a wide, shallow arm-action, in which the fore-arms sweep back beyond the shoulder-line. This has two negative consequences. First, it means that the muscles of the neck and upper torso become the main means of lifting the head clear of the water. Secondly, the wide action of the arms tugs at the neck muscles so that the head is forced backwards. By using a deeper, bent-arm action, the body naturally rises with a minimum of effort and significantly less strain. Using our arms in an effective manner is therefore important for helping us maintain good use.

Practice the appropriate arm-action for the breast stroke by bending your elbows and pulling the arms under your body.

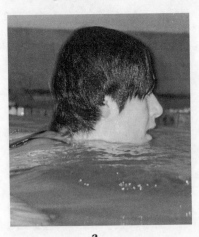 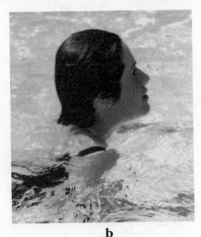

a   b

Fig 4.17
*Breast stroke: the mouth barely needs to clear
the water surface to inhale (a). An excessive lift is a waste of effort (b).*

Notice how this action on its own raises you up sufficiently to be able to inhale without your having to resort to pulling your head back. When your arms remain closer to your body as you pull them back, your head is not drawn back as far. As a result, you not only put less strain on your shoulder girdle, but you can maintain your forward-and-up orientation more easily.

Many breast-strokers retract their head excessively when they come to breathe in, so that their eyes are directed towards the ceiling. But to inhale, your mouth simply has to be high enough to break the surface and be in contact with the air. Any higher is both a waste of effort and reduces stroke efficiency by interfering with the body's streamlining.

When you get into the water, experiment with this aspect of the stroke. Find out for yourself how little you actually need to disturb the head-neck-back relationship in order to raise up your body sufficiently to breathe in. Compare your habitual way of raising your head with a movement in which your face barely breaks the surface. There's a fine line between breathing in adequately and getting a mouthful of water.

The glide in the breast stroke offers the perfect opportunity to discover how *stopping* can allow us to release and naturally extend the body. Keeping the head pulled back interferes with this process of release and extension and impedes the flow and momentum of the stroke. Take advantage of and savour the opportunity of letting go in the glide! This is a liberating experience, enabling us to enjoy a powerful sense of release and natural extension as we move without effort through the water.

Competitive breast-strokers often exaggerate the extension phase of the stroke by incorporating a deliberate stretch into the glide. But what happens to your back if you do this? Over-stretching creates an arching in the lower back and increases tension around the ribcage. Such stretching actually involves a narrowing of the back and compression of the vertebrae – a contraction rather than an extension of the body. This reduces our buoyancy, necessitating more effort to move forward. When we stop contracting, we lengthen and widen automatically, which is all that's required for an effective glide.

Back Stroke

Back stroke is performed with a fluent arm-action combined with a steady up-and-down leg-kick; these require a free-flowing mobility of the hip and shoulder joints. The alternating arm-pull (for propulsion) creates continuous alterations in the body's lateral balance, and controlling body-roll helps to preserve balance and freedom. Maintaining good orientation is the means whereby this can be achieved.

When performed correctly, back stroke can be the most elegant and relaxed-looking of all the strokes. However, if a good head-neck-back relationship is not maintained, it becomes awkward and disorganised. Some swimmers pull their head right back so that their eyes are focussed on a point behind them: this causes the back to arch unduly and water to spill over the face. Others crane their heads forward too far in an attempt to hold their face out of the water. This compresses the chest and puts a strain on the neck-muscles.

Practice the back stroke initially in three stages, to explore the optimum release of the neck-muscles during its performance.

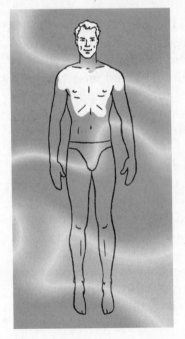

1. *Push off from the pool-side on your back, hands resting by your side. Release your neck muscles, letting your ears submerge, and discover how effectively the water can support your head if you allow it to. Experiment with minor changes in the angle of your neck to see how they can affect the way you float, noticing how holding up the head requires more effort than releasing the neck muscles.*

Fig 4.18

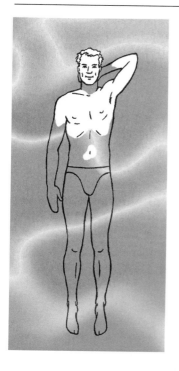

2. *Perform the same procedure with one hand gently supporting the back of your neck. With your hand feel the tone of the muscles in your neck as you experiment with different angles.*

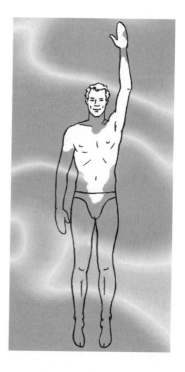

3. *Perform the same procedure, this time with one arm outstretched behind you as you glide. Notice how much easier it is to float with the weight of the arm helping to balance the body along its length. Does this position have any effect on the sensation of release in your neck muscles?*

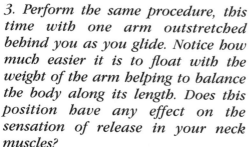

Unlike the breast stroke, back stroke requires taking the arms out of the water and placing them back in. This is a process requiring fine control, and unless performed with awareness and skill can have detrimental repercussions for orientation. The temptation is to arch the back. If we hold our arms stiffly or apply undue force, muscles become taut throughout the body. If the neck in particular is not relaxed, the head will tend to follow the movement of the arm round into the water, pulled both backward and from side to side by the powerful trapezius muscle which connects the neck, shoulders and back. If the backward movement is too extreme, we risk water splashing over our faces. If the sideways movement is exaggerated, we increase resistance to our passage through the water and may disrupt the rhythm of our stroke.

Explore how well you can control the entry of your hand into the water. Whilst neck and arm muscles should remain as relaxed as possible, the hand should be carefully directed into the water, little finger leading. This requires a rotation of the shoulders and a looseness of the neck to allow the head to move smoothly on its axis.

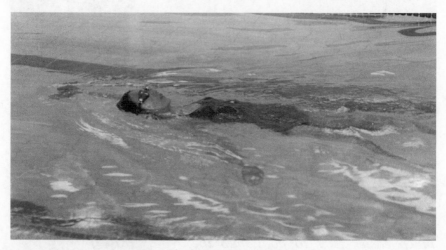

Fig 4.19
Back stroke: the head acting independently of the arms (top); being pulled back by the arm movement (bottom).

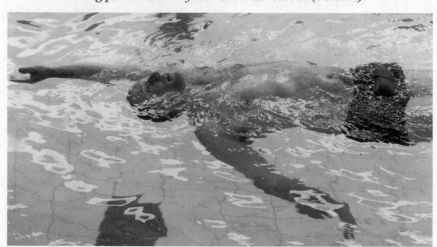

Orientation in the back stroke demonstrates the importance of the "sculling" action which characterises most forms of propulsion in the water. "Sculling" means pushing sideways towards the body with hand and forearm so as to propel oneself forwards on one's front, or backwards on the back. After the arm enters the water, the elbow should drop so that halfway through the underwater phase the forearm can commence to scull. To do this requires a relaxed flexion of the elbow – a rigid arm cannot scull effectively. Furthermore, if the arms flail like windmills or propeller-blades, their very rigidity will cause the strain and imbalance in the stroke that has been described.

Front Crawl

The front crawl (or freestyle) is potentially the fastest and most efficient of the swimming strokes. It is swum in a continuous, flowing action, with the head leading the body through the water like the prow of a ship. When you swim face-down (or prone) you can allow your body to extend naturally and can use your arms with maximum flexibility for propulsion. This stroke offers a good opportunity to explore the experience of release and forward orientation in the water.

Efficient front crawl requires a sensitivity to the changing point of balance along the entire length of the body. The alternate rotation of the arms allows the body and limbs to remain extended as they slice through the water. A useful image is that of a long boat moving forward without a break with a continuous rhythm of propulsion, rather than the push-and-release that gives the breast stroke its characteristic ebb and flow. Longer and proportionately thinner vessels are more streamlined than shorter, broader ones, and this principle applies equally to the way the body lies on the water. In the crawl, the arms, back, and legs are extended. The point of balance of this elongated figure is higher up the body towards the head, creating the potential for greater momentum.

Snatching back the arms in a hasty manner reduces the potential benefit of streamlining offered by the elongated body. To overcome this tendency, it helps to let your forward arm become fully extended (though not hyper-extended) before you start to draw it back. The trajectory of the arms has an important bearing on orientation in the crawl. A bent elbow in the underwater part of the stroke allows for greater purchase on the water, and therefore a more efficient use of effort in propulsion. As the arm breaks the water surface in the so-called 'recovery' phase of the stroke, a high, pitched elbow is important for several reasons. It encourages free rotation of the shoulder and activates the powerful back muscle (the *latissimus dorsi*) rather than putting strain on the arm and shoulders.[4] It allows for greater control and a smoother entry of the hand into the water. In turn an efficient hand entry enables better control of the underwater pull.[5]

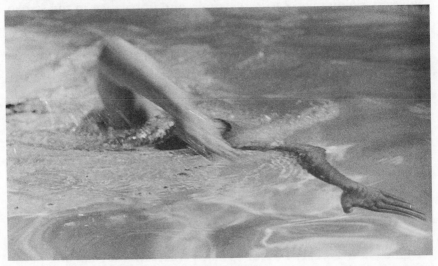

Fig 4.20
The front crawl: both arms, the pulling arm and the recovering arm, are in front of the head for most of the stroke cycle, preserving a forward balance and orientation.

Investigate how the balance of your body shifts when you change the position of your arms from by your side to ahead of you. Explore the feeling by pushing off with your arms by your side: in the shorter stance one feels heavier and cannot travel far. Discover how a longer body position, arms outstretched, enhances

4 Tendonitis of the shoulder, resulting from an incorrect arm-pull, is one of the most common complaints amongst competition swimmers. Research has shown how a bent elbow in the recovery phase greatly minimises the risk of damage.
5 Swimming manuals which mention the *S*-shape of the underwater pull can be misleading. All the swimmer should do is pull back with the arm: so long as the elbow is allowed to bend and flex naturally, it will *appear* to an observer as if the hand in relation to the body describes a curved trajectory as it moves through the water.

*your sense of lightness and flow in the glide, and improves the way
you slide through the water.*

Breathing presents the main challenge to retaining good
orientation in this stroke. Craning the head and shoulders back to
inhale has a particularly adverse effect. Unhurried rotation of the
head and hips is all that's required to lift the mouth sufficiently
above the water to breathe in, and a controlled combination of hip
and head roll is the essence of a fluent, elegant front crawl. You may
believe that the most efficient way to achieve an inhalation is simply
to turn the *head* 90 degrees to the side. Can you do this (even out
of the water) without feeling the pull on your neck muscles? In
practice, a hip-roll which initiates rotation of the torso gives
important assistance to the process. If the hips contribute half the
body-roll, the neck muscles only need to rotate the head half as far.
This creates more time and ease for breath to be taken without
disturbing the balance of head, neck and back.

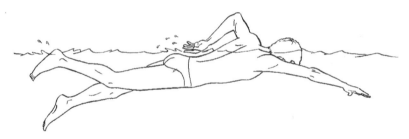

The Hip-roll: *Explore the enjoyable possibilities offered by
increased mobility of the hips in the following way. After
swimming on your front for a few strokes, roll your whole body
over onto your back. Notice how much easier this is if you treat the
body as a unit, instead of twisting your head and neck and letting
your torso follow. Incorporate the sensation of rolling your whole
body unhurriedly into the continuous action of the stroke. As a
rule of thumb, you may find it helpful to think of starting the
outward roll from the hip, and the return roll leading with the
head: think "hips – roll out; head – back in".*

The use of the arms in the crawl, as in the back stroke, also
affects orientation: excessive effort with the arms invariably forces
the head *backward*. Propulsion occurs beneath the water, so
crashing the arms down into the water is both a waste of energy and
militates against the control needed to prepare an effective pull.

Equally, a narrow entry – when the hand enters the water at a point *within* the width of the shoulders – causes the body to wobble unevenly. When swimmers with this tendency first try to bring their hands into the water at a wider point of entry than they're used to, they frequently feel that their arms are entering the water significantly more widely than they actually are.

This is a prime example of what the *AT* calls unreliable sensory appreciation. The faulty arm action has become so ingrained that it *feels right*. When we come to modify it, to start with it feels wrong. Learning the art of swimming is a continuous process of development and refinement of motor skills. We should not, therefore, limit ourselves by relying solely on our feelings: a teacher, external observer, or the aid of photography can be indispensable to the successful accomplishment of the ideas and practices suggested in this chapter.

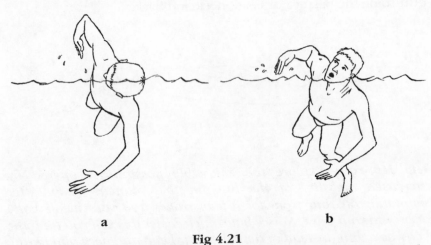

a   b

Fig 4.21
The streamlined orientation (a) is disrupted if one lifts the head and shoulders awkwardly to breathe (b). Note how the lateral hip-roll in (a) helps to maintain a streamlined orientation while turning to breathe.

5. The Art of Breathing

Breathing is the hinge on which the door of life swings.　　Zen Saying

Breathing is vital to the art of swimming. A balanced and rhythmical breathing pattern is fundamental to discovering the joy of swimming and to reaping the full health benefits of being in the water. Problems with breathing, varying in nature and degree, are experienced by swimmers of all levels and abilities. However well you may have mastered the mechanics of a stroke, unless you have learned to co-ordinate the breathing your skills are of limited value. The first step, then, is to become aware of the kind of issues involved.

What happens to your breathing when you swim? Do you hesitate to immerse your face for fear of breathing in water? Is there never enough time to snatch a breath between strokes? Do you dislike the sensation of water getting up your nose so that you hold your breath as long as possible? Does swimming make you unexpectedly breathless despite being reasonably fit?

Whilst many swimmers readily confess to concerns about breathing, others who are not consciously aware of it nonetheless exhibit *symptoms* of anxiety in the way they swim. The anxiety itself, as we saw in Chapter 3, is a stumbling-block to exploring ways of breathing effectively while swimming. The failure to appreciate this means that the need to address *fears* about breathing is often underestimated. It's surprising that they are so rarely addressed explicitly by teachers, swimming manuals and instruction methods. Straightforward, apparently uncomplicated, instructions such as "Turn your head sideways to breathe" or "Breathe between strokes" are virtually useless and offer no enlightenment or comfort to the

123

worried swimmer. Furthermore, they wrongly assume that we will know how to follow such instructions accurately and discover exactly *how* and *when* to take a breath. Such scant regard for breathing is a weak foundation for learning to swim. Even after many years, poor habits and faulty co-ordination of breath acquired in the early stages can persist and mar the experience of being in the water. Learning to co-ordinate breathing with motion is *not* straightforward: on the contrary, it raises complex and important challenges for the art of swimming.

It would be convenient if the only thing breathing required was for one's face to be out of the water. Unfortunately, this is not the case. First, even with our faces held above the water surface, there is no guarantee that we will not *hold* our breath, whether deliberately or unintentionally. In particular, we tend to constrict the free inflow of air, out of anxiety or for other reasons, by involuntarily tightening our diaphragm, the muscle which initiates breathing (see Fig. 5.1). If it were just a matter of nose and mouth being clear of the water, breathing would presumably be no problem in the back-stroke – but it is! In fact, many people find swimming on their back just as problematic (if not more) for breathing as swimming on their front. Secondly, the rhythms available for breathing are different in the various strokes; each stroke raises specific problems requiring different solutions. Whatever the stroke, breathing efficiently in the water is actually a complex activity which requires thought and attention. Inhalation and exhalation need to be finely co-ordinated with the rhythm of the stroke. It takes practice and familiarity to develop a natural rhythm, which varies between individuals and can be freely adapted for different situations.

Fig 5.1 Breathing and the Diaphragm

Breathing requires the motion of the diaphragm, ribs and lungs. The diaphragm is a large dome-shaped muscle which separates the lungs from the stomach and other internal organs (a). When the diaphragm pulls down and flattens (b), it forces the lungs to expand. Air is drawn in through the nose or mouth, which is how inhalation takes place. As air enters the lungs, the surrounding ribcage simultaneously spreads out to allow the upper part of the lungs to expand. A full breath is achieved by allowing the diaphragm to extend downwards so that the lower part of the lungs is filled. *The action of diaphragm and ribs can be impeded by poor use, or even a full stomach.*

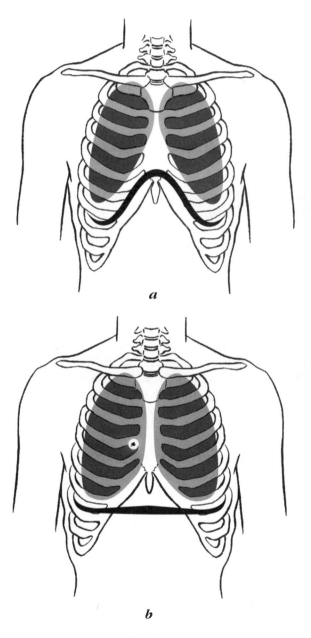

a

b

Fig 5.1

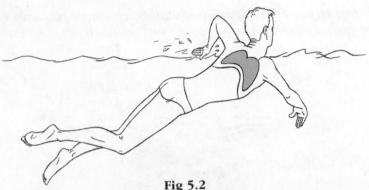

Fig 5.2
Note how an awkardly raised head puts pressure on the lungs ...

When we swim on our front, as in the crawl and breast stroke, our orientation is potentially affected by the need to breathe: in order to take a breath we cannot avoid altering the axis of our head to some degree so that our nose and mouth are clear of the water. This creates an obvious risk of misuse. If we arch the spine or bend our necks backwards at an extreme angle, we not only risk straining them but may find breathing more difficult, because the body-position can constrict the lungs and obstruct the flow of air through the wind-pipe. The art of swimming challenges us to discover the *least* amount of effort needed for us to rise out of the water sufficiently to make an effective inhalation. Good breathing alone enables the swimmer to integrate all the elements of the art of swimming – awareness, orientation, confidence, the effective use of arms and legs, and the overall rhythm of the stroke.

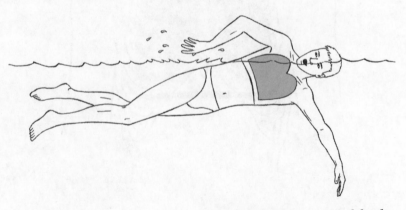

... while maintaining good orientation lets them expand freely into the lower torso.

The need to pay attention to how we breathe is one instance of how being in water can bring about a beneficial awareness of our habits outside the water. If our normal breathing habits are unsatisfactory, as is often the case, they are bound to affect the way we breathe when swimming. Learning to swim can therefore contribute to an increased awareness of breathing difficulties and how to overcome them. Discovering the advantage of breathing with a regular and flowing rhythm in the water has far-reaching consequences for the way we breathe generally. The regular practice of comfortable rhythmic breathing as part of a good swimming style is one way we can improve and strengthen our respiratory mechanism. Doctors often recommend asthma-sufferers to follow a swimming routine for remedial purposes, and Yoga teachers regard swimming as an excellent means of developing a healthy breathing pattern. Meditation and stress-reduction techniques include steady breathing, to produce a calming effect on mind and body. Viewed in this light, the co-ordinated breathing which is part of a fluent swimming style becomes a relaxing and even meditative process for helping us to recharge our physical and psychological energies to approach daily tasks with a new lease of vitality and zest.

Breathing & Health

Breathing is the cornerstone of good health. When we inhale, we take in oxygen, which is not only essential to life but allows us to thrive and grow healthily. If this intake is obstructed we become prone to infection and illness. Exhalation too performs a vital function, expelling stale air from the lungs and toxins from the body. Weak exhalation retards this cleansing process: as well as leaving old air hanging around in our lungs it prevents the full and satisfying uptake of fresh air. As a result the internal organs have to work harder to compensate for the lack of nourishing oxygen and to dissipate the toxic build-up. Common effects of shallow breathing include persistent skin conditions and an unhealthy complexion, poor digestion, and fatigue.

The pressures of modern life mean that most of us breathe in a less than efficient manner – too shallowly, unevenly, and with excessive effort. Breathing disorders such as asthma and emphysema are widespread. Whilst these are usually attributed to environmental factors such as poor air and pollution, they are exacerbated by the effects of misuse. The improvement of overall use through the *AT* is a way of alleviating and sometimes even eradicating such problems entirely. The effect of good use is to enable a healthier way of breathing through freeing up the operation of the diaphragm and ribs. The benefits are numerous – an increase in energy and endurance, a reduction in stress, and improved circulation. The steadier flow of oxygen to the brain also helps to regulate mental functioning. "Take a deep breath" is a way of suggesting that we calm down and allow ourselves to think clearly. In a state of relaxation – when we are asleep, for instance – our breathing naturally tends to be slower and deeper. Regular, unimpeded breathing of this sort has a marked positive effect on our emotional and intellectual well-being.

Equally, we know that our manner of breathing can be affected negatively by strong emotions. Under conditions of stress we breathe faster and more shallowly – in our chest rather than deep into our lower torso. Several automatic reflexes combine to affect our breathing mechanisms when we feel afraid or under threat. One of these is the *startle reflex*, as described in Chapter 3 (see p. 76). Another is the involuntary tightening of the abdominal muscles which accompanies the startle pattern. The contraction of these muscles, a reflex designed as a kind of armouring to help protect internal organs from physical attack, forces the breath to stay fixed in the chest instead of flowing deep into the lungs. Our nervous system also reacts to fear by triggering an increased flow of adrenalin into the blood-stream. Such reactions are characteristic of the *fight-or-flight syndrome*, the evolutionary mechanism which enables mammals to face a potential threat or danger with a burst of unaccustomed strength or agility.

Fight-or-flight is of little value in most situations we encounter nowadays. This unconscious pattern of behaviour, like the startle reflex, is more likely to be an obstacle to efficient functioning under normal circumstances. (Even where special strength and agility are required it may hamper an effective response: martial arts such as Tai Chi stress the importance of full, diaphragmatic breathing for access to vital energy). Our inherited automatic reflexes do not differentiate between situations of danger and moments of emotional stress. Is it really appropriate to react to, say, criticism or embarrassment as if we were facing the prospect of a physical assault? All too often we allow ourselves to overreact *physically* to circumstances in which our *mental* equilibrium is affected. The constant repetition of fight-or-flight reactions is detrimental to both health and clarity of thought. The cumulative effect is to dull our senses and make us tired and edgy. Learning to breathe properly under normal circumstances is a vital step in reversing the tendency to get caught up in this negative cycle.

What are you doing as you read these words? Are you more aware of your breathing pattern? When you think about breathing deeply, do you feel the impulse to sit up or change your posture? Do you recognise the relationship between your the way you are sitting and your breathing? Breathing is one area where the intervention of conscious awareness can have an immediate impact.

Under different circumstances the pattern of our breathing alters automatically. When engaged in high levels of activity we require more oxygen, and our breathing rate increases accordingly. Our hearts pump faster to allow the oxygenated blood in our veins to feed our working muscles. We produce a greater volume of carbon dioxide, a waste gas that has to be expelled from our body by more rapid exhalation. Conversely, when we sleep, our heart-rate falls and our breathing slows down. A similar metabolic change takes place when we swim with our faces in the water: the *dive instinct* has already been described in Chapter 3. It is a factor which naturally affects our breathing rate when we swim. It works to slow down our breathing along with our heartbeat, helping to reduce stress and promote a sense of calmness and well-being. Of course, this can only be experienced if we are confident and relaxed with our faces submerged in the water – another good reason for mastering this requirement of the swimmer's art.

The Alexander Technique and Breathing

You would have found, certainly in Sydney in 1904, that if you'd gone to anybody who knew Alexander and you'd said, "Well, what does this chap do? What's it all about?" they'd have looked at you in surprise and they'd have said "Well, of course, he's the breathing fellow. He's the chap who can really show us what breathing is all about".   Walter Carrington

The *AT* emphasises that good breathing is the natural consequence of good use. It's not a question of trying to control your breathing mechanism. When the torso is allowed to lengthen and widen, we create more space for our lungs to expand. We are all born with the ability to breathe in this free and unrestricted way. Unfortunately we learn habits of poor breathing as we grow up. Observe the gentle and relaxed way in which infants breathe. Their soft tummies expand effortlessly with each inhalation, and release back as they breathe out. Their heads remain poised and pivot freely on their shoulders. The ease they exhibit contrasts starkly with the way most adults breathe: we yawn or strain to obtain a fuller breath by lifting our chests or our shoulders, rather than letting our backs lengthen and widen. And we rarely allow our abdomens to relax.

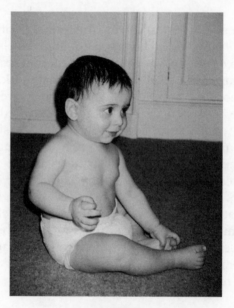

Fig 5.3
Breathing? No problem!

One reason for this is the critical attitude exhibited in our society to the appearance of a relaxed stomach.[1] Other societies are more sensible. The fashionable body-image in contemporary Western culture militates against good use, and consequently

---

[1] The branch buyer of a leading chain of booksellers commented that one of the swimmers on this book's front cover did not have the "right figure for it". Such unquestioning acceptance of an unhealthy stereotype is particularly depressing in the context of the increase in eating disorders in the very young.

against effective breathing. Images of fashion models with unnaturally flat stomachs are pervasive. Men too are encouraged to aspire to an excessively muscular physique, without regard to the distorted body-image which this frequently results in – an overdeveloped torso held up by an uncomfortably narrow waist. Appeals to our vanity can make us feel that we need to hold in our stomachs constantly – though the actual effect this has on our shape is usually imperceptible to others! More importantly, it's a habit which is likely to harm our dynamic balance. It creates a tendency to fix our muscles which affects both our use and our breathing apparatus. The ways in which we are encouraged to pursue "fitness" (see Chapter 2) often compound this tendency. Truly effective breathing requires our diaphragm and ribs to be able to move freely and without rigidity, the numerous different sets of muscles and joints working smoothly in tandem (see Fig 5.1). F.M. Alexander described the sense of ease that good use brings to the process of breathing with the vivid image of "floating ribs".

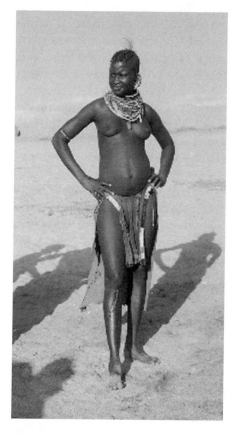

Breathing exercises which require us to hold our breath or otherwise interfere with our breathing mechanism are considered unhelpful in the *AT*. Such exercises, when performed by people whose bodies are already unbalanced by excessive muscular tension and general misuse, are of dubious benefit. How can they encourage an understanding of healthy breathing under normal conditions, with all that this requires in terms of free joints and dynamic muscular balance? Take a person with obviously poor posture – shoulders rounded, back curved, pulling their head back to take uneven

Fig 5.4
a) Turkana women, Kenya.

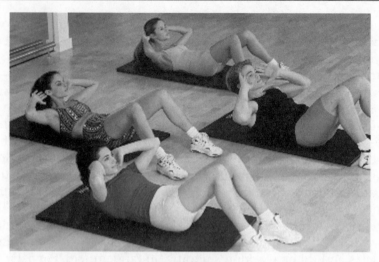

Fig 5.4
b) The crunch.

breaths: when someone in this condition experiences strain in breathing, they cannot alleviate it, let alone eliminate it, with breathing exercises. They may even add to their strain. Gasping for air may be inevitable after holding one's breath for a long time, but it does not encourage regular deeper breathing, and can exert dangerous pressure on the lungs and musculo-skeletal structure. Where poor breathing habits are symptoms of misuse, focussing on breathing in isolation from overall use can only ever be of limited benefit. People with breathing difficulties who are recommended to the *AT* find that their problems can be solved without using any breathing exercises whatsoever.

Most of us are not consciously aware of *how* we breathe. This is an obstacle to improving the way we breathe: the recognition of a bad habit is a prerequisite for effectively changing it. But the recognition in itself is not sufficient to overcome it: the force of habit desensitises our bodies so that to us our misuse often *feels* right. Even when our attention is drawn to poor breathing habits, our own senses are not sufficiently acute to work out accurately what we're doing and how we can bring about beneficial changes. In such instances, the role of a third party, such as a qualified *AT* teacher, can be essential.

What happens when you are told to take a deep breath? Do you push up your chest and shoulders to try and breathe deeply? This action can create the impression that you are breathing fully. But the impression may be false: you may not be aware that the muscular tension in your torso is restricting the free flow of air and that you are only partially filling your lungs.

Genuine improvement in the way we breathe can only arise from a more sensitive appreciation of our overall use, and the application of the principles of good use in our everyday lives.

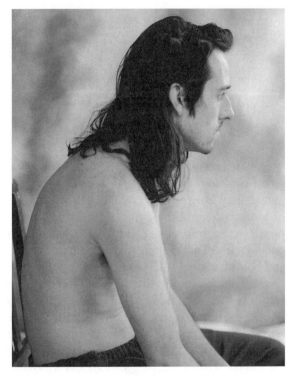

Fig 5.5
Poor use makes for shallow breathing.

Breathing in the Water

How do you read the title of this section? The way you read it may say something about your experience of swimming. If you are confident and relaxed in the water, it simply means *how to breathe when you are in the water.* If you are not, perhaps it conjures up an image of *inhaling water into your lungs* – in other words, choking and drowning!

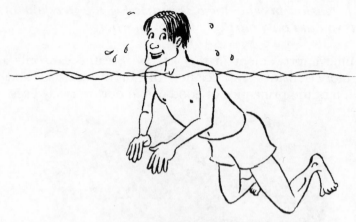

Fig 5.6
*I said "**Breathe** in the water ...*

Being in the water requires us to become aware of our breathing and its ramifications for use. Because we cannot breathe under water, we have to pay attention to our breathing and how it is co-ordinated with the movement of our limbs when we swim. But a number of factors distinguish the way we breathe when in water from the way we breathe on dry land. First, in the water we obviously need to make sure that we avoid inhaling *water* when we take air in – not a problem we encounter on land. Secondly, in a non-aquatic environment we normally breathe in through the nose, which is considered the healthiest way to inhale. The nasal passage, coated with fine hairs, acts as a filter of airborne impurities while regulating the even flow of air into our lungs. When we swim, however, it is more appropriate for various reasons (discussed further on) to inhale through our mouths. Thirdly, swimming requires us to manoeuvre our bodies in such a way that our faces lift clear of the water in order to breathe in. And finally, the inflow of air is one of the things which keeps us afloat, with implications for orientation and streamlining: a steady, controlled inflow and outflow can have a balancing effect on the body; uneven breathing can disrupt the balance.

It's worth emphasising that when we swim a standard stroke, breathing needs to be more regular than under most circumstances. Our breathing rhythm fluctuates constantly as we speak, move, or react to different emotions. When we swim, various factors contribute to create a steadier and more rhythmical pattern.

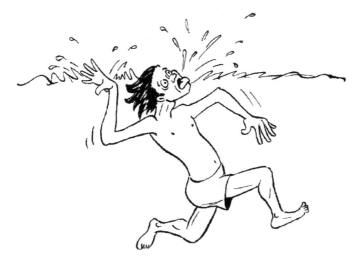

*... not breathe **in** the water".*

We have already mentioned the way the dive instinct slows down our metabolic rate, which can itself have a steadying effect on our breathing. Also, because we usually lie horizontally on the water when we swim, the fact that our body is supported means that we don't need as much oxygen to function, which allows for a lower rate of inhalation. Finally, the water supports our body and cushions the rib-cage, reducing the need for muscular effort when we breathe.

Another factor which distinguishes breathing when water-borne from breathing in other contexts is that when we breathe out, blowing into the water, our senses seem to be more sharply focussed than usual: the sight, sound, and feel of strong exhalation into water can be initially unfamiliar and even alarming. As a result, some swimmers never allow themselves to breathe out with sufficient force, and can be taken aback by how much noise and turbulence seems to be generated when they are encouraged to do so. But it's obvious, when you think about it, that exhalation into water actually needs to be more forceful to achieve the same effect as breathing out into the air: the countervailing water pressure is considerably greater than atmospheric pressure. Some swimmers (such as those who are influenced by Yogic breathing techniques) deliberately exhale more slowly, over the space of two or more stroke-cycles. This reduces the perceptible impact of forceful exhalation, and can stop the swimmer learning an important lesson: the need for a strong outbreath.

It's therefore important to become accustomed to the different sensations aroused by vigorous exhalation into the water. Have fun – blow those bubbles enthusiastically! Even if you think that everyone around can hear you, so what? (In fact they can't – after all, are you put off by the sound of other swimmers breathing?) Fear of causing disturbance is one quite inappropriate reason for holding back from a full exhalation. There are a number of other reasons, often unconscious. The sensation of water pressure against our mouths and noses can feel like a physical barrier preventing the easy outflow of air. This in turn can reinforce a mistaken belief that it's necessary to hold back the breath in the lungs in order to stay afloat. Others may think that the air in their lungs needs to be preserved as long as possible, in case they can't raise themselves up sufficiently or surface in good time to draw a fresh breath. These solutions ignore the need for regular, fresh oxygen. Holding the breath in this way is a sure way of causing panic and hyperventilation.

Case Study 5: Pete – Learning to Breathe

Pete was a moderately strong swimmer who could swim 20 lengths of breast stroke with ease, holding his head up above the water. However, he found that his back became increasingly sore. When an osteopath advised him to swim with his face in the water, he encountered an unexpected problem: he became breathless after just a few strokes and had to stop swimming. He applied for swimming lessons, and his instructor soon detected the source of the problem: although Pete inhaled deeply when his head broke the surface, no bubbles were to be seen when he proceeded into the glide phase with his face under water. The instructor urged him to "blow bubbles", but Pete found the noise disturbing and continued to hold his breath as he had been doing previously.

It transpired that he could not believe that it was "right" to make so much noise under water, and he was convinced that he was the only swimmer in the pool doing so. Only when his instructor demonstrated it did Pete realise that the sound was virtually inaudible to others. He experimented with forceful exhalation until the sound and feel became completely familiar to him. Exhaustion in the breast stroke was replaced by exhilaration at his new experience of swimming for long periods without the sense of strain that had resulted from holding his breath.

In fact, it's noticeable that many swimmers are far more concerned about *inhaling* enough air than exhaling sufficiently. The emphasis should be reversed. Excessive inhalation is itself a major cause of discomfort. If you take in more air than you breathe out, it's inevitable that your lungs will be put under strain: they're struggling to take fresh air into cavities that are already occupied with stale air! You can feel as if you are about to burst. This is one of the main causes of the breathlessness experienced by many swimmers.

Do you find that you complain of exhaustion after swimming a short distance? When you analyse your fatigue, is it that you're moving your limbs with too much effort? Is it because you're poorly orientated and so struggle against the water? Or is it simply that you feel out of breath? For most people, symptoms of exhaustion are the result of an ineffective breathing pattern. Learning to breathe efficiently can be the most important factor in increasing stamina in the water.

Steady breathing also has a calming influence which helps in overcoming all kinds of anxiety. This can be an appropriate starting-

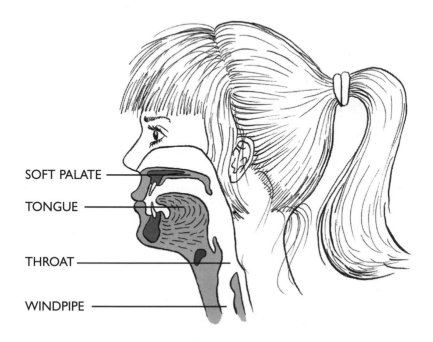

SOFT PALATE

TONGUE

THROAT

WINDPIPE

Fig 5.7
The oral and nasal passages.

point for swimmers who are worried about water getting into their lungs. As we suggested in Chapter 3, it's useful to pinpoint the *source* of fear in order to overcome it. Those who feel such anxiety may find that as their faces go into the water, their ability to exercise control over their breathing is lost. This is often due to the irrational fear that the water will rush into their lungs of its own accord. The discovery that this need not happen can be very liberating. We need to understand and be familiar with the fact that *it only happens if we actively suck water into our lungs.*

This may seem surprising, but it's simply true: we don't have to breathe water in unless we decide to do so! We possess an innate internal mechanism which, if we let it, automatically comes into operation to prevent any water that enters our nose and mouth going further into our lungs. This mechanism is known to speech therapists as the *oral seal*. It operates by gently closing off the path to the throat through the action of the base of the tongue against the soft palate (see Fig 5.7). This allows us, for instance, to breathe in *solely* through our nose – even if our mouth is wide open – by shutting off the oral passage at the entrance to the windpipe. Because of the effectiveness of the oral seal in precluding the unwanted intake of water into our lungs, it's quite possible to inhale air through the mouth without taking in any water – even if our mouth is half submerged below the water. Indeed, this is precisely what allows us to inhale during the crawl without disturbing the flat, streamlined position that is ideal for planing across the water surface.

Discovering the Oral Seal: *In the pool – or in the bath – discover how the oral seal works by inhaling and then lowering your face into the water. Let your mouth open gently without inhaling or exhaling. Notice that even though a small amount of water may come in it will not travel to your wind-pipe. Experiment with how wide you can open your mouth, and explore the effectiveness of this mechanism – it even works when you move your head up or down, or from side to side.*

Because of the way our oral mechanisms operate, it's far less common for water to get into the lungs via the mouth than via the nose. This is one reason why it's more appropriate for swimmers to learn to *inhale through the mouth and exhale through the nose*. Sniffing water up one's nostrils can be a most uncomfortable and disturbing experience! When it happens, little can be done to counteract the water's passage to the lungs – except to exhale forcibly, cough and splutter. However, when we inhale through our mouth, there are at least three points along the oral passage at which we can expel any water that may have inadvertently entered through the mouth, before it gets as far as the windpipe: the lips, cheeks and larynx (the back of the throat).

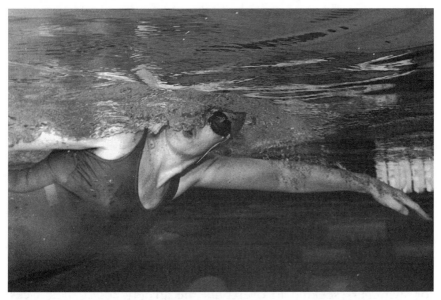

Fig 5.8
The front crawl: as soon as inhalation is taken, the mouth is already virtually submerged – without any fear of water being breathed in.

*Experiment outside the water with these mechanisms. For instance, the **lips**: hold a piece of paper resting against your lips and say "Puff" – notice how the puff of air made by lips alone can push the paper away. Secondly, the **cheeks** – blow as if blowing out the candles on a cake. Thirdly, the **larynx**: notice how the muscles at the back of your throat clench together effectively when you say "Kick". The same muscles can exert strong guttural pressure to expel water or prevent it from entering your windpipe. What happens when you gargle at the back of your throat? Doing this shows that it's quite possible to hold water in your larynx without it slipping into your windpipe.*

Breathing with Ease

The principles of breathing which we have been discussing show that the subject merits far greater consideration, particularly in relation to swimming, than is usually given. In the water, of course, the test of effective breathing is to be able to swim without worrying about it at all! It should feel as if an easy and regular breathing rhythm is integral to the stroke and does not demand any particular effort. Rather like driving a car or accomplishing any co-ordination skill, the initial attention to detail gives way to a greater familiarity with the process that puts all the various aspects of the activity into perspective. The *AT* encourages a flexible approach that allows us to discover what may be appropriate to any situation or activity. In particular, the fact that exhalation in the water requires more force than inhalation is something that needs to be explored in practice.

Ironically, the very effort of focussing intently on breathing can lead to counterproductive tension. In this respect it's worth remembering the lessons of *non-doing* and *redirection*. By thinking of eliminating the ways in which we interfere with effective action, rather than by trying to do it correctly, we can allow our attention to be *redirected* so that automatic habits are not constantly repeated. Attending to the experience of being in the water, rather than trying to control the actual process of breathing, is an example of such redirection. This can be particularly useful for beginners or for swimmers seeking to overcome the anxiety about their faces being immersed in the water. Redirection can be beneficial in any learning activity. A Russian proverb says "We learn to skate in the summer and to swim in the winter". The meaning is that the real learning only takes place when we are *not* concentrating on it. This principle is similar to the *AT* principle of "letting go of the wrong so that the right can emerge" and can be incorporated with benefit into all learning and self-instruction.

Do you worry about breathing out when your face is under water? Instead of worrying about breathing, think about your orientation! Explore the sensation of a streamlined glide with your face in the water. This is a most effective way of helping swimmers to overcome inhibitions about breathing out into the water. By redirecting your attention, you get used to your face being immersed almost without realising it. From there it's a short step to enjoying the sensation of plunging your face into the water. Then, you can explore different ways of breathing out strongly into the water and coming up rhythmically to inhale. Discover your own rhythms in the different strokes. Do you find it more comfortable to breathe out after every cycle (two arm-actions) of the crawl, or after two cycles?

Swimmers sometimes find that the problem is not so much at the point of putting their face *in* the water as when the time comes to bring it *out*. At that point, many swimmers behave as if their head was submerged metres below the surface! Not surprisingly, then, they experience a sense of haste and panic about bringing it out. Snatching the head out of the water often leads to a premature inhalation, usually combined with gulping in an excessive amount of air. Both these actions can cause water to be sucked in to the lungs with all the attendant discomfort. It's important not to rush the inhalation in any stroke, but first to let the water around the mouth and nose run away or be expelled by the lips and nostrils. This short hesitation is not the same as holding the breath, but is a considered, preparatory manoeuvre before breathing in. It provides a space – a split second is enough – in which the necessary mental and physical preparation for the action of inhaling can take place.

Even when the face is submerged, some swimmers exhibit their lack of confidence by breathing out in a jerky or intermittent manner, instead of making a strong, consistent outward exhalation. Because of an automatic tendency to compensate for out-breaths with equivalent in-breaths, such a practice is apt to cause the uncontrolled intake of water. To prevent the potential for mishap, exhalation into the water should be practised so that it is unhurried, even and sustained. This can circumvent a whole range of breathing difficulties. Some swimmers reason that because their nostrils are situated higher than their mouth, it is easier to breathe in through the nose and blow out through the mouth. Outside the water, we usually do breathe in through the nose and out through the nose and mouth. But when swimming, whichever one we choose to breathe *out* of, if we're worried about water getting to the windpipe it's advisable always to breathe *in through the mouth.*

Just as each of the strokes has different breathing requirements, so individuals react differently to their specific challenges. Some swimmers who have an easy relaxed rhythm in the crawl may find difficulty adapting to an appropriate rhythm of breathing in breast stroke. Ask yourself: what areas cause the greatest unease? Why is it easier to breathe in some strokes than in others? Specific issues about the breathing requirements of individual strokes are discussed below. Different factors interfere with easy breathing in the water. At an advanced level, for example, trying too hard to swim fast can produce a lot of tension which has a direct effect on breathing. For instance, the hunched, narrowed shoulders that characterise the competitive model of the breast-stroker at the point of inhalation reduce the potential area available for intake of air, making it harder to take a full breath without effort.

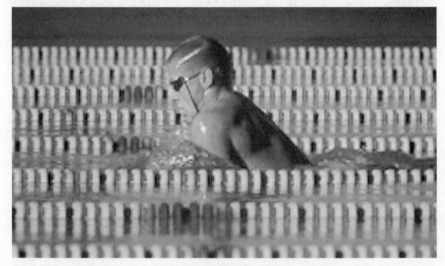

Fig 5.9

A stiff, tense body also impedes comfortable breathing and restricts our ability both to float and to move through the water. The rigid use of limbs and general muscular tension actually encourage us to hold our breath rather than let it flow freely. Unfortunately, competitive training sometimes makes a virtue of such breath-holding: some coaches and swimmers take it to extremes and justify practices that have little bearing on swimming as an art.[2] Holding the breath for extended periods of vigorous activity – whether with full or empty lungs – puts the body under considerable and unnecessary strain. It may improve the racing speed of the sprint-swimmer, but risks damaging his or her lungs and ability to breathe with ease in or out of the water.

[2] Competitive swimming techniques include the practice of deliberately starving the body of oxygen – so-called hypoxic training – in the belief that it magnifies the effects of strenuous activity and thereby provides a more intensive training. Whatever results this practice is alleged to achieve, it is undoubtedly prejudicial to both health and enjoyment.

Conclusion

For Rose [Murray Rose, the Australian swimming champion] swimming was an intensely sensuous involvement, a rhythmic succession of sounds as the hands cut through the water that passed under the body and formed a wave against the side of the face. Rhythm reduces effort. Before a race he would listen to particular music that was close to the rhythm of his stroke. Glen Miller's 'In the Mood' coincided exactly.

Charles Sprawson

While we live, we breathe. The regular rhythm of respiration continues without cease every minute of our lives: to recall the Zen quote at the head of this chapter, life hinges on breathing. Awareness of our breathing is useful because it is always an aspect of the present moment, and awareness of ourselves in the present is the basis of the Alexander Technique. In this chapter we have gone into some detail about breathing processes that are vital to swimming. It makes sense for anyone seeking to learn the art of swimming to give detailed attention to the mechanism and rhythms of breathing, and to apply this understanding intelligently to developing effective patterns of breathing when water-borne. Conversely, paying attention to the requirements of respiration in the water can enlighten us to a new awareness of its function and effect in our daily lives.

We have emphasised that, for the *AT*, good breathing is essentially a function of good use. So long as we are well oriented, with both our mind and musculo-skeletal system in a state of harmonious balance, we are in the optimum condition to breathe in a comfortable and rhythmical way. It's clear that poor breathing habits in daily life can present an obstacle to developing good breathing patterns in the water. But it has also been shown that there are some significant differences about breathing when we swim, which we need to appreciate and incorporate into the way we swim at all levels. In the art of swimming, breathing is itself an art which requires understanding and practice.

Fear and anxiety interact in both obvious and subtle ways with the process of breathing, whether in or out of the water. When we're afraid, we tend to breathe differently, and when our breathing is disturbed, so is our mental equilibrium. The fundamental fear for the swimmer – that of swallowing and inhaling water – can be greatly reduced by familiarity with the mechanism of the *oral seal*.

This is rarely described in the detail that we have gone into here – mainly for the reason that most experienced swimmers and swimming teachers take its operation for granted.

An easy and balanced pattern of breathing is the key to our awareness of the here and now. For those who enjoy swimming, the regular inflow and outflow of breath has both a calming and revitalising power, complementing the beneficial effects of the dive instinct. The combination of the unique properties of water with the principles of graceful movement, woven together into a web of sensuous elegance shaped by the ever-present rhythm of the breath, can be a meditative and magical experience. It takes us beyond the pursuit of fitness and everyday concerns into a realm of artistic grace and harmonious sensation. Reflections on this harmony form part of the theme of the final chapter of this book.

STROKE GUIDE II:
Co-ordinating the breathing

Breast Stroke

In the breast stroke, exhalation takes place as you release into the glide. Pushing the arms forward exerts pressure on the diaphragm, naturally encouraging the expulsion of air from the lungs. Similarly, raising the body up and bringing the arms round in themselves encourage the chest to widen, which promotes an unforced inhalation. At this stage in the rhythm of the stroke, all that's required is for the mouth to be open. Assuming that sufficient air has been expelled during the glide, air will flow in to the lungs without extra effort.

Inhaling generally takes less time than breathing out, and this variance is increased by the fact that breathing out into water requires more force than exhalation into air. Accordingly, the glide in the breast stroke may take many times as long as the phase in which the head emerges above the surface. The length of time you *choose* to take in the glide therefore indicates the speed at which the breath needs to be exhaled. A faster rhythm of the stroke will require a shorter, more forceful exhalation. But if we keep pulling our arms open rapidly, thereby encouraging inhalation with every pull, problems will arise because we're not giving ourselves enough time to exhale fully in the short periods when the arms are in the forward position. The constant pulling back of the arms without sufficient intermediate pause can thus create a tendency to hyperventilate, which is the most common reason for breathlessness in the breast stroke.

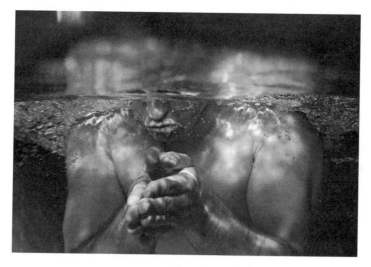

Fig 5.10
The breast stroke: a) push forward, breathe out.

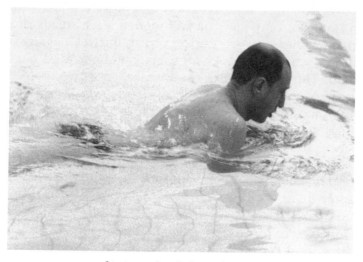

b) Arms back, breathe in.

It is for you to discover your optimum rhythms, and to explore the different possibilities. You can set a rhythm for yourself in advance, for example, by counting to a 4-beat: think "glide" to the count of three, and "up" on the fourth. Explore this when you stand in shallow water: as you push your hands forward, dip your head and exhale into the water. Exhale to the count of 3 while your hands stay together ahead of you, and come up to breathe on the fourth count.

A common fault is to leave the head trailing in the water and then pull it back hastily to breathe. Notice how much easier it is to come up if the head rises as an integrated part of the torso when your arms open and draw back. Note also how the rhythm needs to be adapted when you swim faster and slower. Ultimately, the exact rhythm of breathing will depend on all sorts of factors: your weight, height, speed, orientation – or just the way you choose to swim at the time.

Front Crawl

The challenge in front crawl is to co-ordinate our breathing with the movement of our arms and the accompanying side-to-side roll of the body. Raise your head out of the water too late, and there will be insufficient time to take an adequate inhalation before our arm comes over, forcing our head back round into the water. Twist your head round too soon, and you will interrupt the steady rhythm of the stroke. Either way, we can prevent ourselves making the full exhalation – which is what creates the conditions for a satisfactory inhalation. The crawl, unlike the breast stroke, requires constant movement of the limbs. This is one reason why many swimmers *think* they need to take in far more air than is actually necessary. As a result the flow of the stroke is interrupted, as they hold their face out of the water for an undue length of time.

Experiment with the swift return of the head into the water as soon as the breath is taken, and long before your arm sweeps over in the recovery phase. Notice how much more comfortable this feels compared to the jarring effect of a delayed return, when the shoulder almost collides with the side of your face. You may find it helpful to turn your head so that you look slightly behind *you*

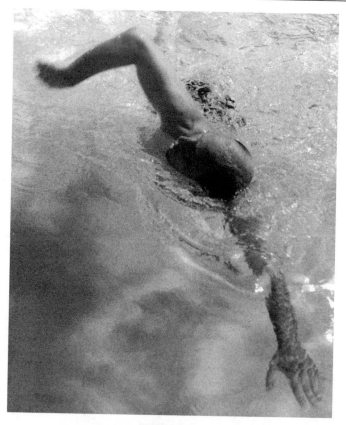

Fig 5.11
Good timing is crucial for breathing. If the face does not swiftly return to the water, the arm may collide with it.

when you come to breathe in. This creates a little more space in which the inhalation can take place.

In efficient front crawl, the in-breath is short and easy, followed by a more prolonged and forceful exhalation. As in the breast stroke, there is no place for the deliberate holding of one's breath. But again, the exact rhythm – or rhythms – will be unique to you. Explore the options and experiment with rhythmical variations, allowing yourself to discover what works or feels best at the time.

Note: Breathing to the side in front crawl: The front crawl is the only stroke in which the head is required to turn to the side for breath to be taken. There's no rule about which side to breathe. For the sake of symmetry swimmers often breathe on each side alternately (*bilateral breathing*). Right-handed people are likely to prefer breathing to the right side, and *vice versa* for left-handers. To avoid confusion, it's a good idea to choose a preferred side and to persist with breathing to that side initially. When you're comfortable with the action to one side, you should practise breathing to the opposite side, so as not to build asymmetry into your body or into the stroke.

Why do swimmers usually find it easier to breathe to one side than the other? One reason is that we quite naturally *incorporate a hip-roll* on the side we are accustomed to breathing on. When instructed to breathe on the unfamiliar side, we usually attempt to do so by turning the head alone. This doesn't allow enough space to breathe with ease; the result is that we pull the head and shoulders further out of the water to compensate. The importance of the hip-roll has been discussed in the section on the Front Crawl in Chapter 4 (see p.121).

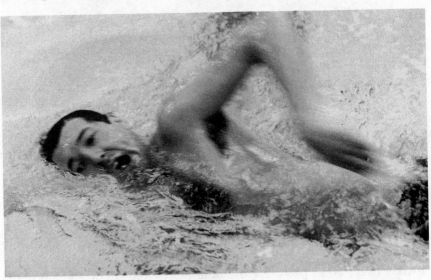

Fig 5.12
Good breathing in front crawl: as in the breast stroke (Fig 4.17), the mouth barely needs to break the surface.

3 Even so, there's no need to inhale water because it's quite possible to retain a vacuum in the nostrils or to blow out through them. Spluttering is invariably caused by alarm, which causes the swimmer to sniff in water involuntarily, rather than taking steps to avoid water getting into the windpipe.

Back Stroke

The most common complaint in relation to breathing in back stroke is that the water seems to get sniffed up the nose into the lungs. How does this happen when the face is resting on the surface out of the water? It usually occurs at the point when the arm goes back into the water. At this point the head tilts backwards, following the trajectory of the arm, and water rushes over the face and into the nostrils.[3] The main reason is that the upper body is not sufficiently free and relaxed for the arms and shoulders to act *independently* of the head and neck muscles.

When back strokers become fatigued and breathless, it's often because they are tightening their neck and abdominal muscles as an unconscious reaction to the anxiety that their faces might become submerged. It's as if they are using their muscles to try to hold themselves up above the surface. The overall tightness of the muscular system prevents the free movement of the ribs and diaphragm, causing the breath to become jerky and uneven. The tensed or fixed body position makes both breathing and floating harder.

By attending to orientation on our back and thereby encouraging the release of such tensions, a virtuous cycle can emerge. We can gain greater trust in our body's buoyancy in the water. This results in greater freedom to move our arms and shoulders independently from the muscles of our head and neck. In turn we acquire increased confidence about being able to breathe when swimming on our back. In this way, we can discover the ability simply to float on our back without anxiety, as well as how to propel ourselves backwards with ease and pleasure.

It follows from this that a relaxed pattern of breathing in the back stroke emerges as a consequence of attention to use. But equally, attention to breathing may itself bring about more relaxed orientation.

Practise different breathing rhythms on your back. Start by selecting one arm to correspond with the in-breath and the other with the out-breath, breathing in and out to the count of "One – two, one – two" as each arm emerges and re-enters the water.

6. In Praise of Water

To plunge into water, to move one's whole body, from head to toe, in its wild and graceful beauty; to twist about in its pure depths, this is for me a delight only comparable to love.

Paul Valéry

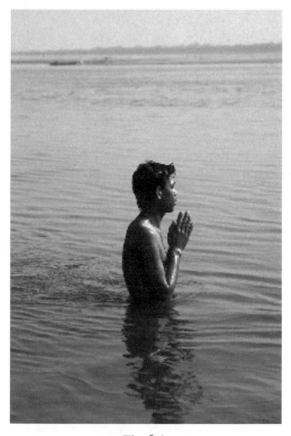

Fig 6.1

Life-giving, cleansing, and endlessly abundant, water has nurtured humanity from the earliest times. When we swim, we are interacting with a medium that has exercised magical associations for people since the dawn of history. In its myriad forms it has inspired poetry, art, literature, music, wonder, exploration, and love. In a world of rapidly dwindling ecological resources, it's a gift to value and cherish. The art of swimming cannot be complete without a profound appreciation of our connection as living beings to the wonderful, unique medium which is intertwined with every aspect of our existence. Water surrounds and embraces our lives with its awesome beauty and variety. We watch it, marvel at it, listen to it, bathe in it, drink it – and swim in it.

According to Ancient Egyptian legend, the gods gave us the gift of water in recompense for giving us a physical body. It was said that through our association with water we become connected to our spiritual nature, and our bodies discover the freedom that our souls have lost. The Hebrews thought of it as a primordial element, present at the origin of the universe, when "the spirit of the Lord moved upon the face of the waters" (*Genesis* 1.2). The ancient Greeks recognised water to be the source of life. They worshipped spirits of the water, and pondered deeply on its spiritual and physical qualities. Their myth, art, poetry and literature reflect on it and celebrate it in all its aspects. More than two and a half thousand years ago, Thales, the first creator of Western philosophical thought identified water as the wellspring of all Being. The poet Pindar praised water in a famous line as "Noblest of all the elements". It was while bathing that Archimedes is said to have made his discovery – immortalised by the exclamation "Eureka!" that marked his insight – that a body's mass can be determined by the amount of water it displaces.

The value of learning to swim is emphasised in many societies and traditions. For the Greeks it was a civilised accomplishment, on a par with learning the alphabet as a basic element of education. They were proud of their ability to swim and dive. Swimming was not viewed as a competitive sport – it did not feature in the ancient Olympic Games – but the Greeks took for granted that it was a skill necessary for self-preservation, for example in the event of shipwreck.[1] The Romans were even more explicit about the instruction of swimming, both for military purposes and for

[1] It's ironic that, despite his extraordinary accomplishments, the one eminent figure in Greek history distinguished by his inability to swim was Alexander the Great.

pleasure: the first mention in history of an "art of swimming" is found in the Roman poet Ovid. In the Jewish Talmud it is considered an obligation – as well as a good deed worthy of respect – for fathers to teach their sons how to swim. In many countries today (including the UK, where it has recently been included in the National Curriculum) children are expected to be taught basic swimming skills by the time they have completed their primary education.

For aquatic creatures like fish, seals, and dolphins, swimming is not an art. But for human beings, relating to water as if it were our element *demands* art. Thinking of swimming as an art encourages us to cultivate the natural affinity that human beings have with the water. It's up to each individual how far we wish to develop that art for ourselves and incorporate it into our lives. Being at home in the water opens up a realm of possibilities which we can hardly contemplate if we are not familiar with the art of swimming. Aquatic activities such as snorkelling, diving, and swimming with dolphins, are exciting ways of expanding our horizons through interaction with water.

The Healing Power of Water

Water is both literally and symbolically the source of life. It's the most abundant substance on the surface of the Earth, covering more than 70% of the planet. It constitutes a large proportion of all living things: about two thirds of a human being's body mass is made up of water. To ensure the efficient functioning of our metabolism and bodily systems, we need to drink it in sufficient quantities every day. Water is a universal solvent, allowing us to assimilate the minerals and vitamins that are vital for strength and health. Insufficient liquid intake even affects the development of bone tissue, ultimately weakening the skeletal framework, reducing its plasticity, and bringing on conditions such as osteoporosis.

The restorative powers of water have been recognised and acclaimed for millennia. Hippocrates, the father of Western medicine, emphasised the importance of drinking for health and had a high regard for water's curative powers. The Greeks prescribed bathing in natural springs as a cure for disease and as a way of increasing vigour and vitality. They filled their town centres with springs and fountains, to give pleasure both to the eye and the ear. Their great medical sanctuaries dedicated to the god Asclepius were established around healing baths and fountains. The Romans went even further, seeking out natural springs wherever they ventured and erecting over them beautifully designed buildings, so that the Roman Bath (like its historical successor the Turkish Bath) is associated with opulence and tranquillity to this day.

Nowadays, water therapies of all kinds are widely used and increasingly popular throughout the world. Spas and hydros are centres for health breaks and convalescence, used in the rehabilitation of a wide range of physical and psychological conditions. Activity in water helps the recovery of wasted and injured muscles; patients who are too weak to move an injured limb without aid may be able to perform a full range of movement in a hydrotherapy pool. Warm baths can help to restore mobility, treat digestive problems, relieve insomnia and promote general muscular relaxation. Cold water is used to lower the body temperature, relieve muscular pains, boost poor circulation, treat skin conditions and reduce inflammations.

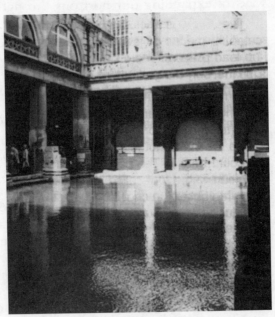

Fig 6.2
Roman Baths.

Whether associated with calmness and tranquillity, or strength and vitality, water has powerful effects on the human mind and spirit. It's well known that the sight and sound of the ocean, of a flowing river, or a cascading waterfall, elicit positive feelings. This is in part due to the actual physical properties of flowing water. At the sea-shore or by the side of a waterfall, there is an abundance of *negative ions*, which has been shown to have a beneficial effect on mind and body. The molecules of the air we breathe carry electrical charges which affect the functioning of cells throughout our body. An excess of *positive ions*, such as is found in most cities, has a fatiguing and debilitating effect.

Even the *sound* of water – a running river or the lapping of waves – produces a measurable effect on our organism. Research has shown that when we listen to the sound of flowing or rushing water, wave patterns in our brain alter in a similar way to when we relax or meditate. Longer exposure to such sounds is used as a way of treating anxiety, tension and depression.

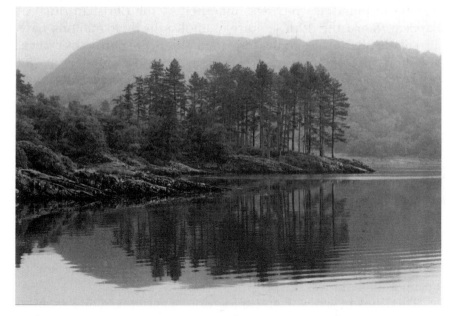

Fig 6.3

Why analyse and treat in isolation all these benefits that water has to offer when water is so abundant? Learn to be alive to the sound, sight and feel of water in all its natural, invigorating and life-enhancing wholeness. Become aware in the water of the inner rhythms of your body. Listen in the silence to your heartbeat as you float motionless. Celebrate the rhythm of your limbs as you swim. Learn to trust water, play with it, and appreciate its tremendous strength. Seek out the currents below the surface, rock gently in swelling waves, feel the water's silky caress on your skin, and submerge yourself in its embrace. In these ways you can discover for yourself the healing power of water.

Reflections on Water

Spiritual and religious associations with water are universal, and water has special associations for many faiths throughout the world. Water symbolises the cleansing of the spirit as well as the body, and this symbolism has frequently been incorporated into religious ritual. Bathing in the holy water of the ancient river Ganges is a religious duty for Hindus. Similarly, there is a religious aspect to bathing in Judaism, which was inherited by the Christian ritual of baptism. Since the 19th century, Catholics in their millions have also made pilgrimages to the sanctified waters of Lourdes in France, and thousands of visitors marvel at the holy springs and the tranquil pools around the Japanese temples to Buddha in the ancient capital of Kyoto.

In the philosophies of Zen and the Tao, the image of moving water is used as a symbol of the flowing, constantly changing nature of life. Water is gentle and yielding, yet possesses tremendous strength. "Nothing in this world is softer than water, but nothing is better at overcoming the hard". Water and its properties are profoundly connected with notions of balance and harmony. The words of the Tao reflect oriental ideas of Yin and Yang, the complementary poles of cosmic force which interact to create the equilibrium of existence. For human beings, awareness of how to bring these elements into balance in our own lives is the key to health and happiness.

This book began with an exploration of awareness, and we have come full circle. Awareness of our self, of the way we stand, move, and breathe, has led us to explore how we relate to our bodies and to the water, and how we choose to lead our lives. We have suggested that the art of swimming can be a source of self-discovery, personal growth and empowerment. A new approach to the water – one which teaches us to be aware of ourselves, to relate it to our organic wholeness and balance, to be at home in the water, to understand and make use of its generous properties, to discover its intimate connections with the rhythms of our life – awakens in us the possibility of a wealth of hitherto unexperienced sensation, and the discovery of unprecedented, indefinable joy.

Come to the waterfall for healing.
Your cousin Water will wash away your negative emotions.
Let the waterfall's mist cleanse and empty you.
Cousin Water will fill you with positive energies and vapours.

Come to the shore of a great lake or sea.
Sit and watch the waves.
See how they move in and out, like your breath.
Follow the movement.

Wonder what shores they have touched.
Imagine the stories of life that they carry.
Time and space will remove itself.
You will become one with Cousin Water.

from
The Healing Drum:
A Book of Native Indian Proverbs

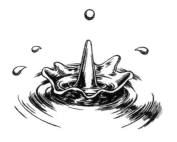

For further reading

The following is a brief bibliography by chapter of books and articles from which we have either quoted or found generally interesting, useful or inspiring. They all illustrate or develop themes mentioned in *The Art of Swimming*. The range of articles available on the Internet is enormous and growing (but the quality varies widely).

Chapter 1. The Wakening of Awareness

The Use of the Self. F.M. Alexander (Victor Gollancz 1992). The key text by the founder of the Alexander Technique.

The Flame of Attention. J. Krishnamurti (Miranda 1983). One of many books recording his thoughts on the art of living.

Zen in the Art of Archery. Eugene Herrigel (Vintage Books 1971). A classic account of Zen through the eyes of a Westerner.

Tensions in the Performance of Music. Carola Grindea, ed. (Kahn & Averill 1987). A collection of essays by experts in various fields.

Chapter 2. Fitness Can Damage Your Health!

Fitness without Strain: a guide to the Alexander Technique. Robert Rickover (Metamorphous Press 1988). A good, readable introduction to the Technique.

Swim for the Health of it. Ernest Maglischo and Cathy Fergusson Brennan (Mayfield Publishing 1985). Top US coach and Olympic swimmer outline health benefits of swimming and provide some useful training programmes.

Swimming for Life: the therapy of swimming. Ronald Russell (Pelham Books/Stephen Greene 1989). Looks at the therapeutic value of swimming for conditions such as asthma, back pain and arthritis, and has a section on swimming for people with disabilities.

On the Internet: "Why Technique matters more than fitness". Terry Laughlin (1994). A series of four brilliant "cyber-coaching" articles by the renowned US swimming teacher.

Chapter 3. At Home in the Water
We are all Water Babies. Jessica Johnson & Michel Odent (Dragons' World 1994). Contains some stunning underwater photographs of infants swimming.
The Water Birth Book. Janet Bolaskas and Yehudi Gordon (Thorsons 1992). A comprehensive guide to pregnancy, labour and childbirth in the water.
Watsu: freeing the body in water. Harold Dull (Harbin Springs 1993). Introduces a new therapeutic method combining principles of Zen, Shiatsu, and Yoga in the water.
Journey into Dolphin Dreamtime. Horace Dobbs (Jonathan Cape 1992). One of many books by a premier delphinologist which explores the relationship between human beings and these extraordinary marine mammals.

Chapter 4. Leading with the Head: Orientation & Balance
Tao Te Ching. Lao Tzu (Penguin Classics).
The Alexander Technique as I see it. Patrick MacDonald (Rahula Books 1989). Thoughts of a well-known teacher the Technique and former pupil of F.M. Alexander.
Haunts of the Black Masseur. Charles Sprawson (Vintage 1993). An unusual blend of the personal, literary and historical celebration of swimming.
Total Immersion: the revolutionary way to swim better, faster, and easier. Terry Laughlin (Simon & Schuster 1996).

On the Internet: "Checkpoints for the crawl" by Kim Carlisle (*Women's Sport and Fitness* 1990). Useful, easy-to-follow tips for stroke improvement.

Chapter 5. The Art of Breathing
Articles and Lectures. F.M. Alexander, ed. J. Fisher (Mouritz 1995).
Thinking Aloud. Walter Carrington (Mornum Times Press 1994). A well-edited series of talks (including one on "Breathing") given by the distinguished Alexander teacher and former student of F.M. Alexander.
Voice and the actor. Cicely Berry (Virgin 1993). Written by the well-known voice coach for professional actors.

On the Internet: "Of Gravity and Air (or is Your Head Attached?)" by Coach Emmett Hines (1994).

Chapter 6. In Praise of Water
The Green Peace Book of Water. Klaus Lanz (Cameron Books 1995).
TAO: The Watercourse Way. Alan Watts (Arkana 1992).
The Healing Drum. Blackwolf Jones (Commune-A-Key Publishing 1995). A book of Hopi Indian poetry.

Useful addresses

Steven and Limor Shaw teach the Alexander Technique and the Shaw Swimming Method (a practical application of the principles of the *Art of Swimming*) to individuals and groups. For details of courses and workshops they may be contacted on 0181 343 0373 or via the Laboratory Health Club, **no.** 2 below, or by e-mail on *100603,1636@compuserve.com*.

1. Society of Teachers of the Alexander Technique (STAT)

The main UK organisation for Alexander teachers. A full list of qualified teachers and a range of information about the *AT* is available. Inquiries (enclosing an SAE) to:

STAT
20 London House
266 Fulham Road
London SW10 9EL

Tel:0171 351 0828
Fax:0171 352 1556

2. Aqua Development Programme (Alexander Swimming School)

The UK's first Alexander-based adult-oriented swimming programme. For details of workshops and other courses contact:

The Laboratory Health Club & Spa
The Avenue
Muswell Hill
London N10 2QJ

Tel: 0181 482 3000
Fax: 0181 482 3688

3. Amateur Swimming Association (ASA)

The UK's official swimming organisation. For information regarding swimming courses in your area contact:

ASA
Harold Fern House
Derby Square
Loughborough   Tel: 01509 234408
Leics LE11 0AL   Fax: 01509 610720

4. Swimming Teachers' Association (STA)

Runs courses in Britain for swimming teaching qualifications nationwide. For details contact:

STA
Anchor House
Birch Street   Tel: 01922 645097
Walsall WS2 8HZ   Fax: 01922 720628

5. National Back Pain Association

Provides information on how to use your body sensibly to reduce back pain.

16 Elmtree Road   Tel: 0181 977 5474
Teddington TW11 8ST   Fax: 0181 943 5318

7. National Asthma Campaign

Providence House
Providence Place   Tel: 0171 226 2260
London N1 0NT   Fax: 0171 204 0740

8. Active Birth Centre

Offers courses, workshops, and practical guidance on all aspects of pregnancy and childbirth, as well as promoting and supplying water-birth pools.

25 Bickerton Road   Tel: 0171 561 9006
London N19 5JT   Fax: 0171 561 9007

9. International Dolphin Watch

A charity which works to protect dolphins and disseminates information and factsheets about the dolphin.

International Dolphin Watch
North Ferriby   Tel: 01482 844468
E. Yorks HU14 3ET   Fax: 01482 634914

Index

Illustrations are indicated by page numbers in **bold** print.